THE 4–WEEK
ULTIMATE BODY
DETOX PLAN

THE 4-WEEK ULTIMATE BODY DETOX PLAN

A Program for Greater Energy,
Health, and Vitality

Michelle Schoffro Cook, DNM, DAc, CNC

WILEY

John Wiley & Sons, Inc.

Published by John Wiley & Sons, Inc., Hoboken, New Jersey

First published in Canada in 2004 by John Wiley & Sons Canada Ltd.

The information contained in this book is not intended to serve as a replacement for professional medical advice. Any use of the information in this book is at the reader's discretion. The author and the publisher specifically disclaim any and all liability arising directly or indirectly from the use or application of any information contained in this book. A health care professional should be consulted regarding your specific situation.

For general information about our other products and services, please contact our Customer Care Department within the United States at (800) 762-2974, outside the United States at (317) 572-3993 or fax (317) 572-4002.

Wiley also publishes its books in a variety of electronic formats. Some content that appears in print may not be available in electronic books. For more information about Wiley products, visit our web site at www.wiley.com.

ISBN-13: 978-0-471-79213-0
ISBN-10: 0-471-79213-6

Printed in the United States of America

10 9 8 7 6 5 4 3 2 1

DEDICATION

I am so blessed with wonderful supportive people in my life. I dedicate this book to Curtis, little Juniper, Mom and Dad, Bob, and Father Ron.

To my beautiful husband and soulmate, Curtis. I celebrate the day you walked through the doorway into my life and every day since then. You are the best thing that ever happened to me and will always be my best friend, confidante, partner, love, and soulmate. I am blessed to share my life with you. Whatever our souls are made of, yours and mine are the same.

To the memory of Juniper. You touched my heart and soul. I will always carry you with me and will never forget you.

To my wonderful and supportive parents, Michael and Deborah Schoffro. Your recognition and nurturing of the writer within me since I was a few years old has immensely helped me in my life. From the early days of writing down my stories for me as I dictated them and listening to my poetry as a child, your love and support have helped me evolve and grow as a person and a writer.

To my sister, for your friendship and fabulous healthy recipes. Your vibrant energy and contribution to my life and this book are greatly appreciated.

To the memory of Monseigneur Ron Synnott. You were always like a father to me, inspiring, motivating, and helping me through some of the most difficult times in my life. Many people do not have one loving father in their life; I was blessed with two. Thank you. You will always have a special place in my heart. You still inspire me.

CONTENTS

FOREWORD

In all of recorded history, humanity has never been engaged in a battle as significant as the one we face today. Never has our future been threatened as severely as it is now. The enemy is not a terrorist organization or a rogue nation seeking global domination; it is the environment we have created —the air we breathe, the water we drink, and the food we consume. We have taken the gifts of life presented to us and poisoned them.

Over the last two centuries, the human race has radically altered this planet and in so doing has radically reduced its own capacity to deal with toxic exposure. The human body possesses an incomprehensible wisdom that we have yet to fully grasp, a wisdom that enables us to heal from a multitude of injuries, illnesses, and traumas. However, our bodies were not designed to manage the magnitude of toxicity we expose them to every day. The result is an epidemic of cancer, respiratory and heart disease, diabetes, allergies, and a multitude of other environmental and physical illnesses. Detoxification, on both a global and a personal level, has become a necessity in our modern world.

My introduction to detoxification grew out of necessity. I was exposed to Agent Orange—considered the most toxic human-made toxin ever produced—on numerous occasions during the Vietnam War. As a result of this exposure, I developed a nerve disease known as peripheral neuropathy that affects much of my body, causing me to limp and limiting the use of my arms and hands. I found no solutions in our conventional medical system and eventually began what has now become my pioneering research and writing in the natural health movement. I learned that my lymphatic system was essential for dealing with toxins in the body and how, by naturally cleansing the lymph and other systems, I could not only eliminate these toxins but also lose weight and alleviate other health conditions at the same time. I am, as far as I know, the longest survivor of Agent Orange–induced peripheral neuropathy. My understanding of toxins and how to overcome them through nutrition and lifestyle choices has saved my life. I have shared this information with millions of people around the world in my *Fit for Life* books.

Michelle shares her compelling story of healing with wisdom and compassion as she gently guides you through this exceptional book. She, too, has lived with the debilitating effects of toxic overload and, through her research and persistence, has created a program that helped her reclaim her life. Michelle's detoxification plan is thorough, covering the intestines, liver, gall bladder, kidneys and urinary tract, lymphatic system, respiratory tract, skin, and blood, while helping to break down fat stores and cellulite—common storage areas for toxins. *The Four-Week Ultimate Body Detox Plan* she presents is comprehensive, but it is not complex. It integrates holistic solutions from both Eastern and Western medicine and reintroduces the reader to all the best things this world has to offer: nutritious food, clean water, living with integrity, and balancing the physical, emotional, and spiritual aspects of our lives.

I am quite familiar on a personal level with the toxic world we live in. So is Michelle Schoffro Cook. Read her book carefully and put into practice her simple, straightforward, common sense principles, and you will be glad you did for the rest of your long and healthy life.

Harvey Diamond

ACKNOWLEDGEMENTS

I would like to thank the many people who contributed to this book, or who supported me as I wrote it:

My soulmate and husband, Curtis Cook: for your unending inspiration, support, and love. To you I am eternally grateful. I will spend eternity expressing my infinite love, admiration, and appreciation for you. Thank you for your tireless effort spent editing this book.

My parents, Michael and Deborah Schoffro: since those first days of writing down my stories and trying to make sense of my poetry, you recognized and nurtured my passion for writing and always encouraged me.

My sister, Bobbi-Jo Meyer, and brother-in-law, Rick Meyer, for your ongoing encouragement to eat a high raw diet that immensely helped my health. Thanks, Bob, for all your great recipes. They make a great addition to this book.

My agent, Rick: for your belief in my work and in me. Thanks for all your hard work and effort to land a publisher for it.

Don and Joan at John Wiley & Sons: for your enthusiasm and belief in this project and vision for its potential.

Harvey Diamond: for contributing the foreword to my book and for pioneering the natural health movement. Thank you for the continued generosity of your time and spirit.

Donna Eden and David Feinstein: for contributing the energy exercises in this book, your willingness to share, and your devotion to increasing the awareness of energy medicine.

My many supportive friends who never stopped believing in me: Carri Drzyzga, Anita Santos, Katerina Taiapa, and Brent and Valerie Sheffler. To my supportive friends who shared their editing skills: Margaret Cinanni, Michele Jarrie, and Darren Francey.

To my many clients for making the days spent in my practice so great, thank you.

To the many other people who offer encouragement and support for all my work, thank you.

CHAPTER 1

How Toxic
Are You?

This sickness doth infect the very life-blood of our enterprise.
William Shakespeare

In this chapter you will learn
   + What toxins are
   + How toxins are affecting your health
   + The many symptoms of toxicity
   + Some of the common sources of toxins
   + What detoxification is
   + How to restore your health to peak performance and vitality
   by cleansing your body of toxic buildup

Imagine waking up without an ache or pain, cruising though your daily tasks with abundant energy, and ending your day with a refreshing night's sleep. Then imagine waking up to do it all over again. Think it is impossible? Think again. An accumulation of toxins can leave you feeling sluggish, achy, heavy, and out of shape. It can also lead to disease in the form of cancer, arthritis, diabetes, allergies, and many other serious illnesses. When you eliminate the myriad toxins in your body, you will greet each day feeling great.

Based on a decade and a half of research and experience, *The 4-Week Ultimate Body Detox Plan* works where other approaches fail. It works by eliminating the source of fatigue, headaches, and joint pain to help you feel great. It works by addressing the causes of minor health problems and more serious diseases such as cancer, multiple sclerosis, diabetes, chronic fatigue syndrome, fibromyalgia, depression, and heart disease. It works by addressing the underlying cause of malfunctioning bodily processes: toxins.

Toxins are substances that disrupt the normal healthy flow within our bodies. Literally thousands of toxins and harmful synthetic chemicals lurk in our food, air, water, clothes, homes, and workplaces. The very things that should nourish our bodies or comfort us are often making us ill. They take the form of foods, cleaning products, beauty and hygiene products, cooking oils, food additives, pesticides and herbicides, industrial chemicals in our air, damaging emotions, sugar, and much more. Take the following quiz to discover the myriad symptoms linked with toxins.

The Detox Quiz

Do you need to detoxify? Take the following quiz to find out. You may be surprised to learn of the many symptoms that are linked to toxins in the body. Score one point for every habit or symptom you have experienced within the last year.

Sleep and Energy
_Tired in the morning or during the day even after a good night's sleep
_Disrupted sleep
_Ordinary activity leaves you feeling exhausted

Mental and Emotional
_Confusion
_Feeling agitated or nervous
_Unexplained feelings of anxiety or sadness
_Excessive anger or irritability
_Mood changes
_Depression
_Memory lapses
_Feeling restless or shaky
_Difficulty understanding new concepts
_Mentally sluggish
_Clumsiness
_Difficulty making decisions
_Negative outlook

Eyes, Ears, Mouth, and Nose
_Itchy ears
_Sensitivity to noise
_Itchy or watery eyes
_Dark circles or bags below eyes
_Swollen or inflamed eyelids
_Bloodshot eyes
_Sensitivity to light

_Sneezing fits or chronic cough
_Runny or itchy nose
_Itchy palate
_Coating on tongue
_Speech problems

Skin
_Dull-coloured, pale, greyish or yellowish
_Loose and flabby
_Wrinkling
_Acne or other blemishes
_Eczema or psoriasis
_Hives
_Cellulite
_Other skin problems

Digestive System
_Nausea or vomiting
_Diarrhea or loose stools
_Constipation
_Belching or gas, especially after eating
_Foul-smelling bowel movements
_Bloating or abdominal discomfort
_Heartburn or indigestion
_Certain foods irritate your stomach
_One or less than one bowel movement per day
_Frequent urination
_Water retention or bloating

Eating Habits
_Have cravings for foods
_Drink alcoholic beverages

_Eat fast foods, packaged or frozen foods
_Drink coffee or tea
_Consume sweets (including any sweetened foods: juices, carbonated beverages, condiments, or desserts)
_Consume white flour products (bread, pasta, cakes, cookies)
_Consume fried foods or margarine

Joints and Pain
_Aching or painful joints
_Joint stiffness
_Headaches or migraines

How did you score?
0–5—Excellent
You are probably experiencing great health. Keep in mind that being symptom-free doesn't guarantee a lifetime of great health. If you are detoxifying regularly, keep up the good work. If not, you may want to consider doing *The 4-Week Ultimate Body Detox Plan* once a year to maintain your health.

6–10—Good
You need to detoxify to improve your health. You will likely find relief from many of the symptoms you experience by limiting your exposure to toxins and conducting *The 4-Week Ultimate Body Detox Plan*.

11+ —Time to Detox
You are experiencing many nagging symptoms that will improve by detoxifying. The energy and effort you invest in healing will pay tremendous dividends. Keep reading—*The 4-Week Ultimate Body Detox Plan* will show you how to get started on the road to incredible health, amazing energy, and an improved quality of life.

Detoxification is the process of cleansing the body of harmful substances, and thereby restoring the body's natural healing ability. This process is accomplished through the use of herbs, foods, juices, aromatherapy, exercise, breathing techniques, and other therapies. Detoxification gives your body a short break from dietary and lifestyle habits that may be wreaking havoc on your health. During this time, you internally cleanse your body of waste products that clog its normal metabolic processes. Even people with minor problems or no visible symptoms often have toxic buildup.

Detoxification is comparable to cleaning your home. Imagine what your bathtub or shower would look like if you did not clean it regularly over twenty, forty, or even eighty years. Yet most people will allow similar conditions to fester in their bodies, without any form of internal cleansing.

Your body has its own ways of dealing with some toxins, but it can be overburdened by the volume and type of toxins found in our modern world. To effectively cleanse your body you must eliminate toxins from your respiratory system, liver, gallbladder, kidneys and urinary tract, skin, fatty deposits (including cellulite), lymphatic system and other detoxification organs and systems. To minimize further toxic buildup you must reduce your exposure to additional toxins.

Using *The 4-Week Ultimate Body Detox Plan*, you will eliminate toxins from your cells, tissues, organs, and organ systems. The results will astound you. You will experience energy you never thought possible and pain-free movement in areas of your body you thought were permanently scarred by pain. You will experience freedom from emotional upheavals, mood swings, and depression. Cravings for less-than-healthy foods will disappear. Your skin will improve and fine wrinkles may recede. Your breathing and digestion will improve, and cellulite will diminish and, over time, may completely disappear.

In years of observing and counselling, I have seen countless people experience the miraculous healing power of detoxification. I am one of those people. When I was only nineteen, my body was suffering from the ravages of toxins. At one point, I was so weak that I could not find the energy to answer the telephone on a nearby night table. While it was not the end of the world that I could not answer the telephone, it was symbolic of how much my life had gone downhill.

It seemed like my life changed overnight. One day I felt on top of the world, jogging, working, and volunteering after school. Then suddenly, I could barely get out of bed. Soon after, I was diagnosed with a serious and rare disorder for which my doctors offered no hope.

After being diagnosed, I was pumped full of prescription drugs to stop my body's own natural processes from working. In a very short time, I could not live without taking the medication upon which my body had become so dependent. My immune system no longer worked. Doctors explained that I could die from a cold or flu or even stress. I was constantly ill, and not long afterward I was diagnosed with chronic fatigue syndrome, which developed because of my damaged immune system.

After seeing countless doctors and specialists, I sought help from the holistic health community. I popped dozens of herbal, vitamin, and mineral supplements. I saw a slight improvement but they were hard on my digestion.

I tried naturopathy, herbalism, acupuncture, and countless other healing modalities. They all helped a bit, especially acupuncture, which started to give me some energy back—enough to spend more time learning how to heal my body of numerous afflictions. I began to wonder whether the diseases from which I was suffering could be linked to toxic buildup. I was shocked to discover the multitude of toxins in our modern world and their insidious presence in the air we breathe, the food we eat, and the products we use.

My body became my laboratory. I experimented with countless detoxification approaches. I chugged olive oil complete with raw garlic and lemon. I fasted on juices. I ate nothing but grapefruit for days. I used herbs and bathed in products that were supposed to pull toxins out of the body. I experimented with every food, folk remedy, fasting method, and healing therapy I read about. I learned what worked and what did not. I discovered the radical misconceptions many authors held about cleansing the body. I quickly uncovered the flaws in their approaches by experiencing terrifying reactions from cleansing too quickly or inappropriately.

Over time, I perfected my approach to cleansing so that it did not entail such drastic diets or therapies. I learned that cleansing did not have to be radical to be effective. It needed to be methodical and harmonious with the body's natural healing mechanisms. I learned that if I tried to cleanse my body while my liver remained sluggish, for example, I would experience headaches, pain, and immense discomfort. I realized that my approach needed to be truly holistic by considering the body as an integrated system, rather than tackling one organ or symptom at a time.

After years of trial and error, I developed an approach to healing that is now the premise of *The 4-Week Ultimate Body Detox Plan*. It is a gentle system that minimizes any reactions. My program consists of simple foods and juices that taste great and require minimal effort to prepare. It uses foods that you can easily find in any grocery or health food store. The cost will be insignificant; your grocery bill will probably shrink while you are on *The 4-Week Ultimate Body Detox Plan*.

The results will astound you as they have astounded me. Once I developed *The 4-Week Ultimate Body Detox Plan*, I started healing more completely than I had in all the previous years combined. At one time, I had almost daily migraines that forced me into a dark bedroom. Now, I do not. The fatigue that plagued me has been replaced with energy and vitality. Many other symptoms that were a regular part of my life are gone. I continue to reap the rewards of detoxification by following *The 4-Week Ultimate Body Detox Plan* regularly.

You will learn some truths about healing your body and afterward your mind, emotions, and spirit. In some ways the body is like a finely tuned and elaborate machine. If you put a piece of scrap metal between two cogs, they will stop turning. If you oil the machine, it will not help. Until you go to the source of the problem (the piece of metal that does not belong there), your machine will never work properly. Similar to the scrap metal that stops the machine from working properly, toxic buildup at the cellular level will be felt throughout the body in the form of disease and degeneration.

If you try to ignore the roots of toxicity, and instead merely treat the symptoms with drugs, you mask the problem and add more toxicity. The symptoms will return and you will be left in a vicious cycle of pill-popping.

The average senior citizen takes eight different pharmaceutical drugs every day. They may take one drug for pain, but it causes digestive upset, so they take another drug for the digestive problems. That drug causes other problems for which they take yet another pill. Soon the pills stop working, so they take stronger medications until they rely on a buffet of drugs just to get through the day. If, instead, they went to the root of the pain initially, they would have no need for so many pills, nor would they experience countless secondary symptoms.

The 4-Week Ultimate Body Detox Plan works on the premise that if you want to heal you must get to the source of the problem. Your doctor may have told you the source of your problem lay in a hormonal imbalance, or inflammation of your joints, or a cancerous tumour. While this is true as far as it goes, it is not the whole story. If toxins build up, the body's healing mechanisms become impaired, preventing them from adequately dealing with naturally occurring cancer cells, excess amounts of hormones, or inflammation.

The buildup of various toxins in the body is a serious contributor to disease and disorder, but one that few people consider. That is because, as we are routinely exposed to toxins, they gradually build up within our bodies. Toxins primarily affect the body at the cellular level, so many people do not get any symptoms at all. But lack of symptoms does not mean perfect health.

Few people ever experience the symptoms of clogged arteries prior to having a stroke or heart attack. Disease may appear to attack quickly and fiercely. Some people experience pain or fatigue or some other negative symptom but only for a short time prior to the diagnosis of serious afflictions like diabetes, multiple sclerosis, lupus, fibromyalgia, or chronic fatigue syndrome.

Other people wrongfully assume that certain symptoms are perfectly normal. Recently, a middle-aged woman told me she had perfect health and that toxins were not an issue for her. Yet she frequently complained of headaches, had experienced menopausal symptoms, and watched her energy plummet on many occasions. While these symptoms are common, they are not normal. They are common symptoms of toxicity and signals from the body that something is wrong. If you ignore these early signs of illness, you do so at your own peril.

Actually, many of the symptoms of illness are also symptoms of toxicity within the body. Illnesses can heal when the body is cleansed properly and rebuilt. The human body is incredible. It is designed to heal—almost anything. Trillions of cells work at lightning speed to remove barriers to health, overcome infection, and heal whatever is affecting your body. That is how broken bones mend and wounds repair. The human body can overcome even the most serious afflictions and trauma when given the opportunity.

In a single second, billions of processes are occurring simultaneously. Things go wrong with the body when we put harmful substances into it, whether we ingest them through food or drink, inhale them in our air, or absorb them through our skin.

You will soon learn the extent of a serious problem and threat to our health and well-being. The human body can withstand minor negligence, but, eventually, it will scream to be heard. It may scream in the form of pain or inflammation, degeneration or organ failure, but it will scream.

When I was seriously ill, I used to believe that my body had failed me. But I discovered that I had failed my body.

Treat your body well and it will take care of you. It has its own innate healing intelligence. Consider the fact that your skin is *totally* renewed every twenty-eight days. You have an entirely new heart in thirty days. Your lungs take seventy days to completely regenerate. So even the most serious affliction should be gone in the time it takes to regenerate an organ. But this is rarely the case. The reason is simple. Your body has specific needs: enzymes, oxygen, nutrients, a proper pH balance, a healthy system of digestion and elimination, electrically charged tissues and cells, healthy emotions, love, and a sense of purpose and fulfilment, among other things. (I will explain more about these elements throughout the book.) If any of these elements are missing, the body will continue with the same diseased pattern.

If your body is burdened with chemicals, sugars, rancid oils, and a lack of nutrients and enzymes at many of your meals, it simply cannot function properly. If every breath you take is shallow and laden with airborne pollutants, your body cannot manufacture healthy cells. If your body cannot manufacture healthy cells, you are vulnerable to ill health. If you slather chemical-laden skin- and hair-care products on yourself, your body cannot use its largest organ of detoxification (the skin) to eliminate toxins. Instead, it is working in reverse, absorbing more poisons into your cells. If you breathe the harmful vapours of chlorine bleach and thousands of other household products, you are exposing your lungs to poisons they were never designed to eliminate.

You may believe your symptoms are the result of a genetic predisposition to some ailment or disease with a name you can hardly pronounce or spell. But these are labels given to malfunctions in the body by Western medical doctors. They mean little or nothing on their own. Consider bronchitis as an example. It is really an inflammation ("itis") of the bronchial passages in the lungs. That is the just the symptom of a problem, but what caused the inflammation? Too often, the Western approach is to provide a pharmaceutical drug for each of the symptoms of a disorder, without thought to the cause of the problem. In addition, these very drugs are synthetic chemicals that stop some process of your body and, at the same time, add further toxins to an already toxic state.

People are not all equally susceptible to toxins. Women are more vulnerable to them for three main reasons. First they are, on average, smaller than men. This lower body weight causes them to become ill from toxic buildup faster. Second, women also, again on average, have more fat in their bodies than men. Toxins have an affinity for fat. When the body cannot handle the quantity of toxins entering it or being manufactured as by-products of bodily processes, it stores them in fat.

That is part of the reason why so many people find it difficult to lose weight. The fat stores in their bodies are serving a valuable purpose: to house toxins, thereby preventing them from causing more damage if they were circulating in the bloodstream or organ systems.

Third, women's hormonal balance is also more delicate than that of men. Many toxins produce hormone-like effects in the body, thereby throwing off this delicate balance.

Children are also more susceptible to toxins than adults. Toxins tend to collect in higher concentrations in their tiny bodies. Also, their immune systems are not fully developed and lack the strength to effectively handle toxins.

Not surprisingly, lifestyle plays a role. If you work with damaging chemicals, are inactive, or breathe toxic fumes regularly, you are more vulnerable to the effects of toxins. If you eat nutrient-depleted food high in additives, sugar, or rancid or hydrogenated fats, you will be increasing your toxic load faster than if you ate healthily.

Exposure to synthetic chemicals also plays a role in susceptibility. Each chemical is different and may react differently in the body. Some are soluble in water while others are not; some break down quickly while others reside in the body's tissues for years. So the specific type of chemical that a person is exposed to may make a difference in how it affects them.

In Chapters 2 and 3, you will learn more about the many toxic synthetic chemicals we are exposed to and their well-documented link to such diseases as cancer, breathing difficulties, imbalanced hormones, lung inflammation, liver damage, high blood pressure, heart disease, diabetes, and much more.

While synthetic chemicals clearly contribute to toxic buildup in the body, they are not the only culprits. There are two main types of toxins: those that come from outside our bodies (exotoxins) and those that come from within (endotoxins). Other external toxins include noise, radiation, electromagnetic fields, weather, altitude, and lifestyle habits. Some internal toxins include emotional traumas and stress hormones, difficult life experiences that get stored in the body, and a loss of a sense of connection to something greater.

It is important that you start thinking of your body as a marvellous creation where millions of functions take place every second. Your body knows how to heal, but it needs your help.

Everyone will benefit from a detoxification process several times per year. People with chronic health concerns should gradually detoxify even more frequently or for a longer duration. *The 4-Week Ultimate Body Detox Plan* easily fits into even the most hectic lifestyle, allowing for an effortless transition into detoxification any time during the year.

I will walk you through my *Ultimate Body Detox Plan*. During the four weeks that make up the program, you will gradually cleanse and purify your body with minimal effort. You will experience few, if any, cleansing symptoms. If you experience any symptoms at all, they will typically be insignificant. They might constitute minimal fatigue or weakness, slight nausea, or a minor headache. If these symptoms appear, I will explain exactly what to do to eliminate them quickly.

Thanks to the natural laws of healing, when you eliminate toxins from your cells, tissues, glands, and organs, the body can resume healthy bodily functions. After we work to cleanse the body, I will show you how to detoxify on mental, emotional, and spiritual levels as well.

The procedures to detoxify the emotions or spirit are clearly different from those used to eliminate chemical toxins in the body. In the following chapters I will address these different approaches and provide you with the tools to start detoxifying. The results of detoxifying are truly remarkable, regardless of your symptoms.

Detoxifying your body, mind, emotions, and spirit has countless benefits. You will observe many irritating symptoms clear up. You can expect that your digestion will improve, your sinuses will clear, your blood pressure may normalize, your bowel movements will regulate, and your hormones will begin to balance. Your energy will soar, and you will see improvements with many chronic ailments.

Your mental abilities will sharpen; you will sleep better, have fewer mood swings, experience a stronger immune system, healthier skin, and lessening of allergy symptoms; and you will feel more capable of living life to its fullest. You may even feel a stronger sense of purpose in your life and a greater connection to the planet and humankind.

It may seem hard to believe that a detoxification program can offer so many rewards, but it is true. I spent years popping vitamins and herbs and trying to eat well, but I saw few improvements in my health. When I focused on cleansing my body, I noticed tremendous improvements quite quickly.

The approach I use to healing is threefold:

1. Cleanse the body of toxins that have built up in the cells, tissues, organs, and organ systems.
2. Reduce further exposure to toxins.
3. Help the body to rebuild through proper nutrition and healing therapies, with particular emphasis on weakened or damaged areas.

This approach sounds simple because it is. Yet it is also powerful and effective. Using *The 4-Week Ultimate Body Detox Plan*, you will learn how to eliminate even the most stubborn toxins from your body. You will also learn how to improve your circulation, so it is better equipped to transport nutrients and remove wastes from your cells. When cells are freed from the burden of excess waste products, they are more capable of fulfilling their purpose. That spells healthier tissues, organs, and glands since cells are their building blocks.

In the chapters that follow, I will take you through the stages of detoxification and healing.

You must first address the toxic load that has already built up in your body. Next, you will eliminate further exposure to additional toxins. Finally, you can start to strengthen any weak areas by providing the body with exactly what it needs to heal fully. I have included short quizzes throughout this book to help you determine the weakest detoxification organs or systems in your body. I will also explain how you can strengthen them to function at their peak.

You will also learn how to maintain the sense of vitality you experience after completing *The 4-Week Ultimate Body Detox Plan* by making small dietary and lifestyle changes. For example, selecting healthier cooking oil can help you sharpen your mental clarity, lose weight, and boost your immunity. By choosing better food storage containers, you can reduce hormonal imbalances.

Foods, herbs, juices, increased oxygen and movement, along with natural healing therapies are the best approach to healing. Restore your body's natural healing instincts by eliminating toxins and you will experience improved health. Henry David Thoreau wrote about the healing effects of nature: "Nature is doing her best each moment to make us well. She exists for no other end. Do not resist. With the least inclination to be well, we should not be sick." If you have the inclination to be well, *The 4-Week Ultimate Body Detox Plan* will walk you along the path to vibrant health and vitality.

In her book *Women Who Run With the Wolves*, Clarissa Pinkola Estés compared the human body to the planet. She declared:

> The body is like an Earth. It is a land unto itself. It is as vulnerable to overbuilding, being carved into pieces, cut off, overmined, and shorn of its power as any landscape. We tend to think of the body as this "other" that does its thing without us. Many people treat their bodies as if the body were a slave. We have only to pay heed to our bodies to know what we must do. The body is not sculpture or marble. Its purpose is to protect, contain, support and fire the spirit and soul within it, to be a repository for memory, to fill us with feeling. It is to lift us and propel us, to prove that we exist, that we are here, to give us grounding, heft, weight. The body is best understood as being in its own right, one who loves us, depends on us, one to whom we are sometimes mother, and who sometimes is mother to us.

In *The 4-Week Ultimate Body Detox Plan* you will learn how to be a better mother to your body—by paying heed to its communication with you via symptoms and by not treating it as a slave any longer. In this way your body will become a more effective repository for memory; it will have a greater, more vital existence and it will be better able to fire the spirit and soul it houses.

In this chapter you learned
- What toxins are and their many sources
- How toxins are affecting your health
- That there are many negative symptoms linked with toxicity
- How to restore your health through detoxificaton

CHAPTER 2

You Are What You Eat and Drink

There is no such thing as a free lunch.
Anonymous,
often attributed to economist Milton Friedman

In this chapter you will learn
- Some of the common sources of toxins in your food
- That synthetic chemicals in your food are linked to aging and disease
- That your body cannot function properly without high-quality fuel
- That sugar in high quantities is not the harmless substance people believe it to be
- How thousands of synthetic chemicals find their way into the foods you eat
- How plastic, yes plastic, in your food disrupts hormones
- That the fats you choose can mean the difference between good health and disease
- The importance of choosing pure water over tap water

Most of us have heard the old adage "You are what you eat," but have you ever considered that you are what you eat, drink, breathe, think, and do? Every food you eat, every beverage you consume, every breath you take, every thought you think, and all the actions you take in life are creating you. This may seem hard to believe but it is true, as you will soon discover in the next two chapters.

Consider that the foods and beverages you consume will be broken down by your body into vitamins, minerals, enzymes, amino acids, fatty acids, and simple sugars, all of which your body will then use as raw materials to create new liver cells, skin cells, brain cells, bone cells, or whatever your body needs to replenish at that time. But what if you eat foods that your digestive tract cannot break down into the building blocks it needs? Or what if the foods and beverages you consumed had very little nutritional value and therefore very few building blocks for healthy cells and tissue? Worse yet, what if these foods and beverages were also laden with synthetic chemicals which your body had to work harder to eliminate but which did not provide the energy your body needs to do that? Even worse still, what if you exposed your body to synthetic chemicals in such vast quantities that it had to struggled to keep you disease-free?

Now consider that the air you breathe determines whether every cell in your body will be adequately oxygenated or whether those cells will have to overwork to eliminate foreign airborne particles or chemicals that your body may not have been designed to handle.

Every thought you think affects your health and well-being. If you think positive, life-affirming thoughts your body will create "feel-good" hormones that will give you greater energy, balanced moods, and overall healing ability. On the flip side, if you think negative, stressful thoughts much of the time, your body will create stress hormones that send messages throughout your body to divert its energy into protecting you from danger—even if that danger is really self-imposed. These stress hormones are beneficial in truly stressful life-and-death situations, but when they are released over long periods of time, they damage your body, as you will soon learn.

The things you do every day affect your sense of well-being. If you work at an office job all day and return home to slouch on the sofa in front of the television, your lack of physical activity will prevent your cells from getting adequate oxygen. Your body's lymphatic system (comparable to a street-sweeping system inside your tissues) will be sluggish and ineffective at removing waste buildup from your body. Slouching in front of the TV will also affect your posture, in turn affecting the alignment of vertebrae, muscles, tendons, nerves, and blood vessels. Over time, this pattern may create back or neck pain as well.

These are just a few of the ways that what you eat, drink, breathe, think, and do affect you. You will learn more about the effects throughout this chapter. You will also learn about the many toxins you are exposed to and the impact they have on your body, mind, and emotions. You will begin to understand how to make healthier choices for your life, the result of which will be improved physical, mental, and emotional health.

THE LINK TO AGING AND DISEASE

Aging is one of life's certainties. Like it or not, we are all aging. It makes no difference whether we are young or old, we are aging. Perhaps the largest factor that determines the speed at which we age is our exposure to toxins. Toxins act as free radicals (highly reactive molecules that bind to and destroy cellular compounds, even our genetic material) in our bodies. We encounter toxins in our foods, beverages, air, cosmetics, personal hygiene products, home, workplace, car, stressful thoughts, emotions, and more. Our exposure to toxins affects all aspects of our health.

Let's talk about free radicals for a moment. They are derived from our environment, foods, and beverages or are produced within our bodies. They include radiation; air pollutants; fungicides, pesticides, and insecticides; anaesthetics; pharmaceutical drugs; over-the-counter (OTC) drugs; petroleum products; excessive sunlight; fried, charbroiled, and barbecued foods; alcohol; coffee; sugar; chemical solvents found in furniture, carpets, paint, and office equipment; and stress hormones.

Free radicals have numerous effects in our bodies. The way they damage cell walls may predispose people to heart disease and stroke. The way they disrupt internal mechanisms of cells may lead to genetic damage and a predisposition to cancer. They cause reduced immune function leading to increased susceptibility to infection, cancer, and rheumatoid arthritis. They speed the aging process and destroy the proteins in skin, which leads to a loss of tissue elasticity and increased wrinkling.

You are exposed to many different toxins in an average day. The food and beverages you eat and drink are often full of sugar, synthetic chemicals, and hydrogenated fats. You may be eating excessive amounts of trans fats or animal protein that have a negative impact on your kidneys. The soap, skin-care and hair-care products, and perfumes and colognes you use are typically loaded with toxic chemicals you absorb through your skin or lungs. If you are frequently stressed out, your body secretes hormones that wreak havoc on your body over time. If you use pharmaceutical or over-the-counter medications, they often contain chemical fillers, heavy metals, and substances that have to be filtered by your body's detoxification systems. Depending on your lifestyle, you may be adding further toxins to an already overloaded system. These may include household cleaning products, building and furnishing materials in your home, cigarette smoke, recreational drugs, or excessive alcohol consumption.

Our bodies have developed sophisticated detoxification mechanisms over many thousands of years to eliminate most of the naturally produced toxins they encounter on a regular basis. The Industrial Revolution and its resulting synthetic chemicals found in places such as food, water, soil, air, household and workplace materials, and medicine have created a new dilemma for the human body. Our bodies simply cannot handle the onslaught of synthetic chemicals we throw at them. We may be able to handle some of these toxins but over time, the large amount consumed, drunk, inhaled, or absorbed by the average person greatly exceeds his or her body's capacity.

YOU ARE WHAT YOU EAT AND DRINK

Let's say that you just bought a beautiful new vehicle. It looks fabulous and you are so proud to own it. What would happen if you used poor-quality gasoline as fuel? It contains residue and useless by-products of the drilling and refining processes. Over time, that gorgeous new vehicle would get poorer and poorer gas mileage, it might start having engine knock and excessive wear, and eventually the engine would likely malfunction.

Your body is similar to a vehicle in that it requires high-quality fuel to function properly. By high quality, I am referring to food that Nature provides that is loaded with plentiful amounts of vitamins, minerals, fibre, enzymes, and many other building blocks to great health. These are the things holistic health practitioners are talking about when they refer to "nutrition."

Before we discuss what high-quality fuel for humans consists of, let's take a look at the standard North American diet—something that is more adequately referred to as "no-trition." The average person eats large amounts of fatty foods; animal protein; sugar; and packaged, prepared, or fast foods. While this may be average, it is by no means normal. To help you understand what I am suggesting here, let's take a look at these dietary excesses and shortcomings one by one.

A SWEET LIFE?

To misquote Shakespeare: sugar by any other name would taste as sweet. Sugar may taste sweet but it is hardly the harmless substance many people believe it to be, especially in high doses. The average North American consumes 149 pounds of sugar every year. Stack 149 one-pound bags up in your kitchen and you'll have a good idea just how much that is. You will barely have room for anything else.

"Not me," you may quip, or "I couldn't possibly eat that much sugar, someone else is making up for me." While that may be possible, it is not very likely. Even if you rarely consume desserts, you may be surprised to learn some of the ways that sugar sneaks into your diet. Of course there are all the obvious places, such as soft drinks (the average North American drinks 486 ten-ounce cans of soda pop every year; each one contains about eight teaspoons of sugar), ice cream, cake, and cookies.

Nancy Appleton, author of the best-selling book *Lick the Sugar Habit*, identified some of the following lesser-known sources of sugar. What about that hamburger you ate last weekend? Shockingly, the meat was most likely injected with a sugar solution to prevent it from shrinking. Many meat packers feed sugar to animals prior to slaughter. This "improves" the flavour and colour of cured meat, at least according to the food industry. The average bottle or package of "juice" may not even contain a single drop of juice from any fruit. More likely, it is loaded with sugar, colours, and artificial flavours to give it that "natural" fruit juice flavour. The breaded coating on most prepared foods contains sugar, and salmon is usually glazed with a sugar solution before being canned. Sugar is used in the processing of luncheon meats, bacon, and canned meats. It is also found in such unlikely items as bouillon cubes and dry-roasted nuts. Peanut butter and many dry cereals (even many of your so-called healthy favourites) contain sugar. This one may shock you: some salt contains sugar! Almost half the calories found in most condiments, such as ketchup, come from sugar.

Refined sugar, in the large doses we consume, may be one of the worst poisons we put into our bodies. Sugar blocks your body's immune response for between four and six hours. That means your body is more likely to fall prey to the thousands of viruses, bacteria, and other infectious diseases present in our environment and in our bodies during that time. Although we are quick to blame those pesky pathogens, we rarely look to that decadent triple chocolate cake or that scrumptious sundae. How could anyone fault something that looks and tastes so sweet?

The proper functioning of white blood cells is integral to a healthy immune system. Research shows that both sugar and alcohol consumption inhibit white blood cell activity. The amount of sugar in one soft drink will stop white blood cell activity within thirty minutes and normal activity will not resume for four to five hours. You are more vulnerable to bacterial and viral infections after consuming sweets because your white blood cells are unable to function properly to fight these foreign invaders.

Our sugar addiction is having detrimental effects on our health. Plenty of studies link sugar consumption to cancer, hormonal disruptions, arthritis, osteoporosis, cataracts, and many other degenerative diseases, the list of which is massive.

In one study hamsters were fed diets high in sucrose (refined white sugar). Some were also fed calcium supplements in their food. The calcium made no difference—the hamsters developed osteoporosis, regardless of how much calcium was in their food. Researchers credited high sugar consumption as the *primary cause* of osteoporosis in this study.

Sugar makes the pH in your body very acidic. Countless studies link acidic body chemistry with disease. The same diseases that thrive in an acidic body rarely exist if the body is returned to a more neutral pH. In the case of osteoporosis, your body recognizes that acidic blood can cause damage to your arteries, organs, and central nervous system. In its wisdom, your body recognizes that drawing calcium from the bones neutralizes the body's pH. This mechanism is fine for short-term amounts of acidity but it is a contributing factor to osteoporosis over the long term.

Sugar also contains over sixty synthetic chemicals left over from the many processes it endures to transform a thick, fibrous, brownish stalk of sugar cane into the white crystalline substance we call sugar. Although you will not find bleach, deodorizers, and all kinds of other garbage listed on the label, you would find it present in small amounts if you took some sugar to a laboratory for analysis. Not to mention that government regulations insist that white sugar must have all the vitamins and minerals removed so that it can be labelled "sucrose." These nutrients and fibre "waste" products are the substances that help your body digest sugar without massive blood sugar fluctuations.

Pseudo-Foods and Chemicals in Disguise

Forget aspartame and saccharin and the myriad other artificial sweeteners—they are worse than refined sugar. Countless studies show that they are powerful health destroyers. Of course, the research that is conducted by the manufacturers of these chemicals never indicates any link to health concerns. Research done by independent organizations that do not have a vested financial interest in these synthetic sweeteners links these products to many serious health problems, including birth defects, brain tumours, menstrual irregularities and premenstrual syndrome, migraines and headaches, epilepsy and seizures, psychiatric disorders, blindness, and even death. Which studies would you believe?

Artificial sweeteners are synthetic chemicals your body has to break down, chemicals your body may find it impossible to break down, chemicals your body was never designed to digest. The manufacturers of these products know this information and twist it with slick marketing campaigns to make you think that something that travels through your body undigested (and therefore has no calories) is good for you. According to them, foods sweetened with these chemicals are just a fabulous way to eat sweets without paying the price. Wrong. Wrong. Wrong.

No matter what the slick advertisements or product packaging might suggest, there really is no such thing as a free lunch. Nature in its infinite wisdom designed your body to perform many functions on the food you ingest as part of the overall digestion process. You will learn more about these processes later in this book, but for now you need to know there are many organs that interact with every morsel of food you ingest. Each one is designed to break that food down to extract any goodness it offers and eliminate the leftovers. If something cannot be broken down, your body wastes energy in a futile effort to do its job. These chemical substances clog your body's natural detoxification mechanisms and make them less effective.

Imagine if every day you poured bacon fat down the drain of your kitchen sink. The drainage pipes were designed to handle water and small particles of food. If you keep pouring bacon fat into the drain, it will clog and become ineffective at allowing water through—the very substance it was designed to handle.

The same is true of your body. It was never designed to handle the artificial chemicals used by the food-processing industry. You may be surprised to learn that more than three thousand additives and preservatives are found in our food supply today[1] before that food reaches your table. It is inundated with artificial colours, flavours, flavour enhancers, bleach, texture agents, conditioners, acid/base balancers, ripening gases, waxes, firming agents, nutrient enrichers, preservatives, heavy metals, and other chemicals that find their way into your food.

Even before that food is processed, your food has been sprayed with pesticides, herbicides, and fungicides, most of which are linked to health problems in humans.

An apple a day might have kept the doctor away prior to the industrialization of food growing and preparation. According to research compiled by the United States Drug Administration (USDA) Agricultural Marketing Service, Pesticide Data Program, today's apple contains residue of many toxic chemicals used during the growing process. In only one category of chemicals, known as organophosphate insecticides, this federal government agency found residue of many different neurotoxins: azinophos, methyl chloripyrifos, diazinon, dimethoate, ethion, omethioate, parathion, parathion methyl, phosalone, and phosmet. That doesn't sound too appetizing, does it? Neurotoxins are substances that medical research has proven to be toxic to the brain and nervous system of humans.

You may be thinking, "Well, in minute amounts maybe pesticides are okay." Think again. The average apple is sprayed with pesticides seventeen times before it is harvested. A study by the United States Environmental Protection Agency (EPA) identified more than fifty-five pesticides that can leave cancer-causing residues in food.[2] According to the Natural Resource Defense Council, the use of pesticides has risen more than tenfold since the 1940s. Currently, over 1.2 billion pounds of pesticides are used in agriculture every year in the United States alone.[3]

Dr. Patricia Fitzgerald cites a study by the Pesticide Action Network in her book *The Detox Solution*, showing that more than fifty million pounds of fungicides, herbicides, insecticides, and soil fumigants were applied to farmland in California alone in 1998.[4] One year. Every year over 2.5 billion pounds of pesticides are dumped on crop lands, forests, lawns, and fields.[5]

Pesticides are not water-soluble. That means they are not easily washed off apples or any other food. The same is true once they are in your body—they are hard to eliminate. Fat-soluble pesticides are actually attracted to the fat stores in your body. Don't have much fat? Your body will start to hold fat to prevent these toxins from running rampant throughout your bloodstream. In your body's innate wisdom, it recognizes that these substances cause damage if they travel through your blood so it attaches them to fat in your body. That spells weight gain and difficulty losing weight at best. At worst, these dangerous neurotoxins attack your body's organs, tissues, brain, and nervous system.

Consider one well-known pesticide that was banned in Canada and the United States three decades ago—DDT. It is still being manufactured and exported around the world to appear in our imported foods.[6] According to Dr. Fitzgerald, "Each year, the EPA performs a study of the chemicals found in human fat tissue samples. DDT continues to be found in 100% of the tissue examined."[7]

Dr. Jozef Krop, a leading environmental medicine physician in Canada, asks a poignant question in his book *Healing the Planet One Patient at a Time*: "When the food we eat is grown in nutrient-poor soil, watered with acid rain, sprayed with pesticides, and treated with food additives, and when the water we drink and the air we breathe are also contaminated, is it any wonder that chemicals have been detected in human blood and fat tissue?"

Not only is today's apple not adequate to keep the doctor away, it is more likely to keep the doctor on call. Virtually every food item that is grown using commercial (non-organic) farming techniques contains these or other neurotoxins.

And what if that apple is processed into a frozen apple pie or the fast-food apple pies we consume in droves? There is a good chance that this apple will transform from a nutritious food into a toxic food-like substance we call "food." Any of several thousand chemicals will be added to this apple during the many stages of processing.

Have you ever noticed that the incidence of food allergies and sensitivities seems to be higher than ever? I believe that many people are reacting to the potentially thousands of chemicals used in the growing and processing of foods, rather than the foods themselves. Of course, some people are reacting to the food. But, considering that the average person eats 124 pounds of food additives every year,[8] toxic chemicals definitely play a role in our health.

Farmed fish, particularly salmon, is one source of an especially nasty group of chemicals: PCBs. You may have read about the high amounts of polychlorinated biphenyls (more commonly known as PCBs) found in salmon. Salmon isn't the only culprit. PCBs have shown up in other types of fish and in chicken, beef, pork, eggs, and even milk. This is quite an alarming discovery because research showed that PCBs were (and still are) powerful carcinogens and as a result were banned in the 1970s in both Canada and the United States. Some government organizations claim that trace amounts of PCBs are fine. But one organization's trace amounts are another's poison. Consider that Health Canada and the United States Food and Drug Administration argue that foods with less than two thousand parts per billion (ppb) of PCBs are fine to eat. On the other side of the coin, the United States Environmental Protection Agency states that levels as low as fifty parts per billion are associated with an increased risk of cancer. Yikes! So if the experts can't agree, what's a person to do? Limit your consumption of animal products and, of course, limit your consumption of farmed fish. During *The 4-Week Ultimate Body Detox Plan* you'll be avoiding these items anyway. The break will do you good.

Recent research shows that food colourings cross the blood-brain barrier.[9] There is a lock-and-key type of mechanism in your brain that allows some substances (such as nutrients) to go into the brain while preventing damaging substances from attacking the brain. This is referred to as the "blood-brain barrier." The term "barrier" creates a false sense of security, because chemicals such as food dyes trick the brain into allowing their entry, putting them in a position to do harm to perhaps the most delicate organ in your body.

Consider one very common and well-known food additive: monosodium glutamate, better known as MSG. This pervasive chemical is added to food to enhance its flavour. It is frequently found in Chinese food, as well as in the following food ingredients, so don't be surprised if you don't see it labelled as MSG on ingredient lists:

autolyzed yeast
calcium caseinate
gelatin
glutamate
glutamic acid
hydrolyzed protein
hydrolyzed soy protein
monopotassium glutamate
sodium caseinate
yeast extract
yeast food
yeast nutrient

Many people react within forty-eight hours of ingesting even a small amount of MSG, making it sometimes difficult to trace back to the originating food item. Symptoms commonly suffered include headaches, dizziness, nausea, diarrhea, burning sensation of the skin, changes in heart rate, and difficulty breathing. According to Dr. Patricia Fitzgerald, "Ingesting MSG over the years has also been linked with Parkinson's and Alzheimer's."[10]

A Cup of Java

I know this is probably the last item you want to see in a book about toxins. After all, what if it means giving up your morning (or mid-morning, afternoon, or after dinner) coffee? Some detox programs on the market will tell you coffee is good for you. Truthfully, coffee beans that are shade- and organically grown, properly harvested, stored, and roasted, and drunk in moderation may even have some beneficial properties (for people who are not sensitive to coffee or don't have an illness that is aggravated by it). The amount of pesticide-laden coffee that is consumed in North America is the primary problem. Most often, coffee is grown in third-world countries where toxins such as DDT are used. *Coffea arabica* tends to be from Central or South America while *Coffea robusta* is usually grown in Indonesia or Africa. Also, states Dr. Patricia Fitzgerald, "the farming methods used to grow non-organic coffee are rapidly altering ecosystems, especially in the rainforest."[11]

Coffee is a source of caffeine, which in large amounts is linked with cardiovascular disease, fibrocystic breast disease, cancer, and behavioural problems in people. It is also linked with ulcers and heartburn. In sensitive individuals, coffee can have detrimental effects on psychiatric disorders.

Women who take oral contraceptives have an impaired ability to eliminate caffeine from their bodies, making them more susceptible to the effects of caffeine (even in moderate consumption).

For non-sensitive people, drinking shade- and organically grown coffee, even one to two cups per day, is typically fine.

Paper filters used in the extraction of coffee from ground coffee may be a culprit in the negative effects associated with coffee. Numerous studies found dioxin residues in bleached paper coffee filters. Dioxin has been linked to suppressed immune function, decreased vitamin A in most organs, decreased vitamins D and K, and bleeding in babies. Dioxin also seems to negatively affect the thyroid hormone regulatory system and has carcinogenic potential.

Various chemicals such as trichloroethylene, trichloroethane, ethyl acetate, and methylene chloride are used in many decaffeination processes to extract the caffeine from coffee. One exception to this is Swiss water-processed decaffeinated coffee, which is the best option if you drink decaf coffee. Not enough research has been carried out on effects of the chemicals used to decaffeinate coffee, so it is best to go the route of Swiss water-processed to avoid consumption of these potentially harmful substances.

Alcohol

Alcohol taxes the body's detoxification systems because it has to be processed by the liver, which reduces the liver's capacity to perform the other five hundred functions it has to do. Excess alcohol is stored in the liver, and binge drinking can lead to cirrhosis of the liver and hepatitis. "Research has also shown an association between alcohol consumption and cancers of the mouth, esophagus, liver, and breast."[12]

Even moderate drinking in people with slightly impaired liver function can be a problem, not to mention that even in people with no known alcohol-related problems, alcohol can decrease the liver's ability to detoxify the body. As you learned earlier, alcohol inhibits white blood cells, preventing them from performing their important tasks to keep your immune system strong.

When Plastic Gets in Your Food

Just what is plastic doing in a chapter about foods and beverages? Toxins found in plastics and plastic wraps frequently find their way into our foods. Once there, they "mimic the estrogens that are linked to breast cancer and other hormone-related illnesses."[13] According to Leslie Crawford in her February 2004 article, "Containing Plastics" in *Alternative Medicine*: "Many of the chemicals used to make and treat the plastic we wrap and bottle our food in may be carcinogenic, hormone-altering, and, at the very least, a cause of allergic reactions ranging from skin irritations to breathing problems. What's more, a growing body of studies shows that many of these same toxic chemicals are migrating directly into our food."[14] Activist groups such as Greenpeace and government agencies such as the United States Department of Agriculture (USDA) and the Centers for Disease Control and Prevention (CDC) are closely watching some of these chemicals. Unfortunately, no long-term studies have been conducted on the effects of plastic exposure on humans, even though it remains the most widely used packaging material in North America.

The range of plastic-type substances in our food supply ranges from plasticizers (which soften hard plastic), polyvinyl chloride (PVC) (which is hard plastic), and others. Dozens of animal studies conducted in the last few years demonstrate that many of these plasticizers are harmful to pregnant mice and their babies. One plasticizer in particular, bisphenol-A (BPA), is linked to chromosomal (that is, genetic) abnormalities. According to research reported by Leslie Crawford, "Exposure to the chemical, which creates hormonal imbalances, resulted in everything from high rates of spontaneous abortions to decreased sperm counts in male mice and early onset of puberty in female mice." While that does not necessarily imply the same effects for humans, it is cause for concern.

According to Ned Groth, a senior scientist for Consumers Union, in Yonkers, New York, when plastic is exposed to high heat or harsh soaps or when plastics are simply used repeatedly over time they can degrade and make their way into our food.[15]

Crawford cites several plastics that are culprits to be wary of: vinyl or PVC, polystyrene (PS), and polycarbonate (PC). PVC is used in cling wrap in grocery stores and delis, bottles used to store cooking oils, and some water bottles. It contains substances that are suspected carcinogens and hormone disruptors. Polystyrene is found in disposable plastic cups and bowls and opaque plastic cutlery and usually contains substances that are also suspected carcinogens and hormone disruptors. Polycarbonate is used for clear plastic baby bottles, five-gallon water jugs, clear plastic "sippy cups" for babies and children, and clear plastic cutlery. Many plastics of this kind contain unknown plastic ingredients that are linked with hormone disruption.

According to some experts, all the studies that show plastic is safe for use in the food industry have been conducted by the plastic industry itself. If you are unsure, I go with glass containers.

Health Risks on the Barbie

Because barbecuing does not involve cooking meat and vegetables in oil, it might seem like a healthy alternative to stove-top frying. Sadly, this is not the case. "Drippings from chicken, beef, or fish can splash down on hot coals during barbecuing and create a carcinogen called benzopyrene. This chemical is returned to the food through smoke."[16]

The high temperatures involved in barbecuing food can create mutations in the food, especially if the food becomes charred. These "mutagen" compounds have been linked to cancer and birth defects.[17] Dr. Patricia Fitzgerald cites studies that found when PhIP (a substance produced in high-temperature cooked meat) was fed to rats, tumours developed in the animals' mammary glands. She also cites a German study of nine hundred women that showed those "women who ate plenty of charred and grilled meats had a two-fold greater risk of breast cancer than female participants who rarely or never consumed these foods."

Hydrogenated and Trans Fats

Even if you don't know much about hydrogenated fats or trans fats, you would probably agree that they sound like some kind of experiment gone awry in a science fiction movie. These fats seem like some experimental food produced in test tubes by evil scientists that come to life at night and start attacking everything in sight. Well, that's actually not far from the truth.

Hydrogenation is a process using high temperatures to change the structure of fat molecules from a liquid to a solid. The food industry benefits from this unnatural process because it prevents the oils from becoming rancid. People respond positively to the marketing campaigns that tell you the product will last longer. But what is the human cost of this experimental food substance? Hydrogenation turns healthy fatty acids (cis-fatty acids) into harmful ones (trans-fatty acids). Cis-fatty acids, which are sometimes called essential fatty acids, trigger healthy fat metabolism in the human body. They are critical to a healthy brain and nervous system, immune system, organs, tissues, and cells.

After a fat has been chemically altered to become a trans-fatty acid, it no longer offers any of these benefits. Instead, the human body does not even recognize it as food. It treats trans fats as toxins and searches for dumping sites in the body—fat stores. In some cases, trans fats get dumped into organs, like the liver, which usually cannot filter all of them over long periods of time.[18] Trans fats can also clog the liver and prevent healthy fatty acids from being absorbed from healthy foods. I refer to trans-fatty acids as "plastic fats" since they really do not resemble food any longer.

The melting point of trans-fatty acids found in today's margarines and most prepared and packaged foods is 46 degrees C. These fats do not melt or break down at body temperature (37 degrees C).

Stick margarine is up to 30 percent trans-fatty acids while shortening is up to 50 percent of these harmful fats.[19] Most oils found on grocery store shelves contain trans fats as well. This is because of the high heat used to extract the oils from nuts and seeds during the manufacturing process.

Cooking oils to high temperatures, as in home cooking or industrial cooking, can cause the healthy fats to turn into trans fats. That includes most fried foods, potato chips, commercial salad dressings, baked goods, candy bars, breads, cookies, and chocolates, all of which can contain between 30 and 50 percent trans fats. If you check the ingredient list, you will typically find items such as "partially hy-drogenated oil" or "hydrogenated vegetable oil" or "shortening or vegetable oil shortening." These all indicate the presence of trans fats. Within the next few years, Canadian and American laws will require the amount of trans fats or hydrogenated fats to be listed on the label.

Cold-pressed oils or extra-virgin olive oil are better choices than commercial cooking oils, margarine, and shortening.

Water, Water Everywhere, Is it Safe to Drink?
You might think Samuel Taylor Coleridge had transported himself from the eighteenth century into the present time using a time-travel machine when he wrote, "Water, water, everywhere, nor any drop to drink." Our water supply has increasingly become contaminated with various pollutants and shows no sign of improving in the near future. According to Dr. Patricia Fitzgerald, "The Environmental Working Group and Natural Resources Council have jointly estimated that one-fifth of the American population drink tap water containing lead, fecal material, toxic waste and/or other pollutants."[20]

You might be surprised to learn exactly what is found in your water supply. Over a hundred studies on tap water worldwide found that pharmaceutical drugs often escape water treatment. These studies found cholesterol reducers, painkillers, chemotherapy drugs, antibiotics, beta blockers, Prozac, and anti-seizure medications in tap water *after* it had been purified by city and town water treatment facilities.[21]

One of the main substances found in water is chlorine. It is not the safe stuff most people believe it to be. We are so accustomed to hearing that our water supply is chlorinated that we think nothing of it. Yet in numerous studies conducted by Harvard University in conjunction with the Medical College of Wisconsin, researchers linked the consumption of chlorinated water to 15 percent of all rectal cancers and 9 percent of all bladder cancers.[22]

Even if you purify your drinking water, you are at risk of absorbing chlorine through your skin. In a study published by the *American Journal of Public Health* and conducted by the Massachusetts Department of Energy researchers found that 50 to 70 percent of exposure to water pollutants in adults occurs through the skin.[23] That's right—you absorb water pollutants through your skin while showering or bathing. Dr. Patricia Fitzgerald cites a New Jersey study that showed elevated breath levels of chloroform in people hours after they had taken a shower. She adds, "Taking a shower exposes you to as much as six times the chloroform (a toxic compound in chlorinated water) through steam as you would absorb from drinking treated water."

And what about that lovely bleachy smell we attribute to pool water? You guessed it: swimming in chlorinated water is another way that we absorb toxins through our skin. If you own a pool, ozone is preferred to toxic chemicals to purify the water.

If you live in an older home that has lead pipes or lead solder used on copper pipes, the lead can leach into your drinking water.

"In a classic study, John Yiamouyiannis, Ph.D., compared cancer death rates in the largest fluoridated and non-fluoridated cities in the U.S. The rates were similar in both cities before fluoride was first introduced in 1953, but then rose noticeably in the study areas where fluoride was used. Indeed, a researcher at the National Cancer Institute has concluded that fluoride causes more cancer deaths than any other chemical—blaming it for an estimated 61,000 cases of cancer in 1995. Other scientists warn that additional sources of fluoride (toothpastes, pesticide residues, etc.) in combination with treated water can result in toxic levels of exposure and a weakening of teeth and bones."[24]

In 1996, over 45 million pounds of chemicals were discharged into surface waters, including lakes and rivers that supply drinking water.[25] By 2000, that amount had risen to 260 million pounds[26]—

six times as much! This ongoing and voluminous amount of water pollution threatens our water supply. If you are counting on city water filtration systems to eliminate these toxic waste products, think again. Most city and town water purification facilities are not capable of eliminating the thousands of different chemicals now readily found in water.

According to research conducted by the American Chemical Society, exposure to chemicals by inhaling air in and around the shower is up to a hundred times greater than by drinking water. As you will learn in the next chapter, the chemicals that you inhale in the shower are not the only ones to be concerned about.

Drugs, Drugs, and More Drugs

Move over, Rolaids and Tylenol. Step aside, Tums and Seldane. If you spell relief D-R-U-G-S you may wish to reconsider.

Drugs are made of synthetic chemicals that must be filtered by your liver, kidneys, and other detox organs. They also deplete vital nutrients required for detoxification. Basically, they add to your body's toxic burden while reducing its capacity to eliminate them.

I am not suggesting that you discontinue taking any medications that your doctor has prescribed. Doing so can be very dangerous. I am asking you to rethink the necessity to pop a pill for everything that ails you. After all, what did people do only a hundred years or so ago, before there were prescription and OTC drugs?

Repeated use of medications can weaken your detoxification organs and your body's ability to detoxify. Drugs do not eliminate the underlying causes of the symptoms people take them for; instead, they merely mask them. The cause of the original problem that was covered up by drugs may rear its ugly head somewhere down the road in a much nastier form.

Harvey Diamond, the best-selling health book author of all time with his book *Fit for Life*, adds: "When the cleansing efforts of the body are suppressed with drugs, the level of toxicity increases until other organs become affected as well, not only with the toxins already in the body but also… with the added toxicity of the drugs that are administered."[27]

The *Journal of the American Medical Association* reported, "Every year more than two million Americans become seriously ill and 106,000 of them die, all from prescription drugs."[28] The study to which they are referring clearly indicates that these deaths are from the CORRECT use of prescribed medications, *not* from incorrectly mixing medications or taking them incorrectly. That means that more than *one million* people died in the nineties from the correct use of their prescribed drugs. Drug side effects are the third highest cause of death.[29] The pharmaceuticals that millions of people turn to for relief from pain, inflammation, and other symptoms are not only causing side effects, they are actually killing many people.

By some estimates, six thousand people die every year from "simple" non-steroidal anti-inflammatory drugs (NSAIDs). The side effects of these drugs contribute to congestive heart failure, kidney disease, suicidal depression, cataracts, ulcers, macular degeneration, hearing loss, tinnitus, memory loss, fatigue, and liver disease. Whew! You might want to think twice before popping a painkiller.

The average senior citizen, over age sixty-five, takes thirteen prescription drugs per year. You guessed it: they start out taking one drug for one problem but need another medication to counter the side effects of the first drug, and so on, and so on. That number does not even include the number of over-the-counter medications people are taking. Research has not been conducted to determine all the possible harmful effects of taking so many toxic pills at once.

Medications deplete many of the vitamins and minerals needed to ensure proper detoxification channels in your body. Over-the-counter pain relievers such as Aspirin, Advil, Aleve, Tylenol, and the countless others on the market deplete your body of vitamin

C, folic acid (vitamin B9), iron, zinc, and many other nutrients. All these nutrients are needed for efficient detoxification and to build healthy cells and blood.

All medications need to be filtered by your body's detoxification systems. These detox systems may already be overburdened by the various toxins mentioned earlier. What happens when the organs don't have the nutrients they need to do their jobs because these vitamins and minerals were displaced by drugs? You guessed it: toxin overload. So what's a tired and toxic body to do? *The 4-Week Ultimate Body Detox Plan.*

In this chapter you learned
- Some of the most common sources of toxins are found in your food in the form of pesticides, food additives, sugar, trans fats, and other toxic chemicals
- Synthetic chemicals in your food have been linked to aging and disease
- Plastic in your food disrupts hormones and is linked to cancer
- Medications add a burden to the detoxification organs while depleting your body of vital nutrients needed for efficient cleansing

References

1. Patricia Fitzgerald, *The Detox Solution* (Santa Monica, CA: Illumination Press, 2001), p. 70.

2. Fitzgerald, *The Detox Solution*, p. 28.

3. Fitzgerald, *The Detox Solution*, p. 29.

4. Fitzgerald, *The Detox Solution*, p. 28.

5. "The Importance of Detoxification." Informational Brochure. Advanced Nutrition Publications, Inc., 2002.

6. Fitzgerald, *The Detox Solution*, p. 28.

7. Fitzgerald, *The Detox Solution*, p. 28.

8. "The Importance of Detoxification."

9. Jacqueline Krohn Frances Taylor, *Natural Detoxification: A Practical Encyclopedia*. (Port Roberts, WA: Hartley & Marks Publishers, Inc., 2000), p. 115.

10. Fitzgerald, *The Detox Solution*, p. 73.

11. Fitzgerald, *The Detox Solution*, p. 78.

12. Fitzgerald, *The Detox Solution*, p. 79.

13. Fitzgerald, *The Detox Solution*, p. 82.

14. Leslie Crawford, "Containing Plastics." *Alternative Medicine*, February 2004, p. 72.

15. Crawford, "Containing Plastics," pp. 72, 116.

16. Fitzgerald, *The Detox Solution*, p. 83.

17. Fitzgerald, *The Detox Solution*, p. 83.

18. Siegfried Gursche, *Good Fats and Oils* (Vancouver: Alive Books, [year of publication?]), p. 14.

19. Gursche, *Good Fats and Oils*, p. 15.

20. Fitzgerald, *The Detox Solution*, p. 42.

21. Fitzgerald, *The Detox Solution*, p. 42.

22. Fitzgerald, *The Detox Solution*, p. 44.

23. Fitzgerald, *The Detox Solution*, p. 42.

24. Fitzgerald, *The Detox Solution*, p. 44.

25. "Detoxification." Informational Brochure. Advanced Nutrition Publications, Inc., 1994.

26. "The Importance of Detoxification."

27. Harvey Diamond, *The Fit for Life Solution* (St. Paul, MN: Dragon Door Publications, Inc., 2002).

28. Diamond, *The Fit for Life Solution*, p. 61.

29. Michelle Cook, "How Do You Spell Relief—Drugs or Natural Remedies?" *Health 'N' Vitality*, February 2002, p. 20.

CHAPTER 3

You Are
What You Breathe,
Think, and Do

Search for the cure within the cause; the body itself
is the best healer.
Plato (c. 429–347 B.C.)

In this chapter you will learn
- The effects of what you think about all day long
- How unmanaged stress creates toxins in your body
- That there are thousands of toxic chemicals in cigarette smoke,
  including second-hand smoke
- The many sources of air pollution
- That your household cleaners are not as safe as you may think
- Chemicals in your hair-care and body-care products and
  cosmetics are rapidly absorbed through your body's largest
  detoxification organ

YOU ARE WHAT YOU THINK AND FEEL

Most people are already aware that almost every day a new miracle compound is found in fresh fruits and vegetables and that people who eat large amounts of produce reap the health benefits of doing so. We also know that eating junk food results in more than just biggie-sizing of your clothing. It clogs arteries and is linked to cancer and many other degenerative diseases. Have you ever noticed that the miracle compounds and nutrients discovered by research scientists are never found in packaged or fast foods, or milk, or beef, or pork? They are found in fruits and vegetables. So we know that eating more fruits and vegetables will have a positive effect on our health, but have you ever stopped to consider how your thoughts and actions affect who you are? If you are like most people, this thought has probably never crossed your mind.

A sage once claimed, "Man is what he thinks about all day long." What do you think about during your days? Do you think about how exhausted you are? Do you find life dull and boring? Or perhaps you think life is difficult and overwhelming. Does your attention regularly revert back to the pain in your body or the emotional dissatisfaction you feel? These thoughts are not as innocent as you may imagine. On the contrary: they are the building blocks of your body, mind, and spirit. They are what you will become.

Researchers Robert Jahn and Brenda Dunne at the Princeton School of Engineering found in their studies that a large number of test participants could influence microscopic physical events at a distance, including the output of computerized random number generators. The only tool at their disposal for affecting the "randomness" of the numbers generated was their mind. The participants in the study were able to "will" events to happen in a specific direction merely by focusing their conscious minds.[1]

The results of this study are profound. They suggest that things we previously believed were random events, or coincidence, can actually be affected by our thinking. What is more impressive about this study is that the people's thoughts affected a computerized system. Most people currently believe that inanimate objects such as computers are not affected by our thinking. This study proves them wrong.

But what are the implications for us? The study suggests that a person's thoughts and expectations can affect the outcome of a situation. Consider that with respect to your thoughts. Do you constantly tell yourself how tired you are? how you don't have enough time or energy or money? how you ache? or how life is a burden? These thoughts are creating your tomorrows. Surely it is easier to affect the outcome of expectations on life experience than it is to affect a computer. What if every day you wake up believing that life is difficult? Perhaps you are helping to fulfil your own beliefs.

Conversely, what if you begin to expect the best from life? What if you start to believe that you can make significant changes in your life that will improve your health, energy, immune system, and overall feeling that life is great? If you change your thoughts, you can change your life. If you allow yourself to feel positive emotions, you can create profound change in your life.

Biologist Glen Rein at the Institute of HeartMath, in Boulder Creek, California, conducted a study of people who entered a state of heartfelt appreciation or unconditional love, what he referred to as "heart consciousness." He found that these people could actually alter the winding and unwinding of DNA (genetic material) in solution. It did not matter whether the participants were holding the DNA in a test tube or not. By allowing their hearts to be full of positive and loving emotions, the participants in this study were able to affect DNA in a test tube! When the same people held loving feelings in their hearts, their heart rhythms became extremely coherent. Their electrocardiograms (ECGs) were analyzed by sophisticated frequency-analysis software. Whenever they held the loving, appreciative thoughts, the same unique coherent rhythm pattern found in their ECGs could also be measured in the trees growing outside the HeartMath facility.[2]

That people's thoughts could affect the life force of trees may seem more like science fiction than reality. But more and more studies by leading scientists, quantum physicists, and world-renowned researchers are *proving* that our thoughts and feelings do have significant effects.

If you maintain an open mind and accept the validity of these findings and their immense implications for improving your health, you will likely find these studies empowering.

The research that proves the power of our thoughts and emotions continues. Crime rates in various cities in Africa were studied during the periods just prior to, during, and after large groups of advanced Transcendental Meditation (TM) instructors were conducting large meditation sessions. Crime rates fell to very low levels during these times, where prior to the arrival of the TM groups, the rates had been high in all the cities studied. After the group departed, the crime rates rose again to the baseline rates.

If thoughts during meditation can affect crime rates, then surely our thoughts can affect what happens in our own lives and in our own bodies. You may wish to think twice before participating in road rage or other destructive habits. You may also wish to take time out of your day to meditate, which you will learn in Chapter 7.

One of the world's foremost authorities on heart disease, Dr. Dean Ornish, found that his strict dietary and lifestyle approach to overcome heart disease helped some people, but there was still a "missing link" for others in whom he witnessed fewer improvements. When he began delving into the stifled emotions behind his patients' illness, his success rate soared. In his book, *Love and Survival*, Dr. Ornish writes, "I am not aware of any other factor in medicine that has a greater impact on our survival than the healing power of love and intimacy. Not diet, not smoking, not exercise, not stress, not genetics, not drugs, and not surgery."[3]

Because of the importance of emotional cleansing and the power of self-love to heal our bodies and improve our lives, it is a component of *The 4-Week Ultimate Body Detox Plan*. We will explore ways to shift your thoughts and emotions for emotional cleansing in Chapter 7. Proust stated: "The real voyage of discovery consists not in seeing new landscapes but in having new eyes." Throughout *The 4-Week Ultimate Body Detox Plan*, I will ask you to have new eyes, to stop seeing things in the same way as you always have. I will ask, and already have been asking, you to open your mind, expand your awareness, and approach life differently than you have in the past.

You are being asked to change any negative thoughts and expectations to positive ones to help with both emotional and physical cleansing. You are also being asked to approach the dietary and lifestyle changes you will be making over the next four weeks with a positive attitude. If you begrudgingly undertake the detox regime with a bitter and resentful attitude, the stress hormones and negative energy you will be creating will affect your results. Your body will feel more like a battle zone than a peaceful place where life improvements create profound results.

If you have never tried detoxification, you have a great opportunity to expand your horizons and discover greater potential for your body, mind, and soul. If you have tried other detoxification programs, you have the occasion to explore the possibilities of delving deeper and cleansing your body more thoroughly than ever before. Along with that exploration comes the chance to experience life differently.

YOU ARE WHAT YOU BREATHE AND DO

Your body is intricately affected by the things you do, whether you lead an active or inactive life, the environments in which you spend time, the products you use to clean your home, the personal hygiene products and cosmetics you use, the quality of the air you breathe—the list is endless.

One of the things we do twenty-four hours per day is breathe. It is, for the majority of the population, a virtually unconscious act. It is a necessity, and yet we may take it for granted that every time we inhale, the air will contain the gases we need to maintain a functioning body. Air pollution is changing this reality in many parts of the world. Breathing can be dangerous to your health.

There are many sources of air pollution. Some are natural, such as smoke from naturally caused forest fires, dust from soil, ash from volcanoes, meteorological phenomena, natural gas, terpenes (a class of unsaturated hydrocarbons found in plants), and ammonia from biological decomposition. Most air pollution is human-caused. There are petrochemicals from transportation, such as buses, cars, planes, and transport trucks. Fuel combustion factories, refineries and power plants, as well as industrial manufacturing facilities, spew out toxic chemicals in droves. Waste and waste disposal processes create air pollution. Aerial and land spraying of farms, electromagnetic and electrical emissions, and chemical dumps all create air pollutants.[4]

In 1996, more than 418 million pounds of chemicals were released into the ground and over one billion pounds of chemical emissions were pumped into the air.[5] In 2000, more than four billion pounds of chemicals were released into the ground and almost two billion pounds of chemical emissions were pumped into the atmosphere. Yikes! Our planet, not to mention our bodies, simply cannot be expected to deal with such a massive amount of neglect and abuse.

According to the National Research Council, no toxicity data are available for 80 percent of the chemicals currently in commercial use,[6] while 95 percent have not been tested for their long-term effects on human health. A number of reasons could account for this, including the fact that over seventy thousand chemicals are currently in commercial use. At the same time, experts estimate that to conduct a single long-term animal study of just one chemical substance may take two to three years and cost approximately $1.5 million.[7]

It is generally accepted among scientists who study the pathways of pesticides and solvents in the body that these substances travel through the bloodstream and eventually end up in the body's fat.[8] This poses a problem for ongoing or high levels of toxic exposure. Where do all the synthetic chemicals go? Fat, fat, and more fat. I believe that increasing levels of obesity and overweight are linked partly to increasing chemical exposure. You will learn more about reducing fat stores that house toxins and contribute to weight problems later in this book.

Up in Smoke

Unless you've been living in a cave or have been in denial for the past twenty or so years, you are probably well aware of the dangers of smoking cigarettes. But did you know that one in five deaths in the United States is the result of tobacco use, according to the American Cancer Institute?[9] This could be because there are over four thousand known toxins in cigarettes[10] in addition to nicotine.

Ralph Klein, Alberta's premier, a smoker and a man known for his bluntness, recently stated, "Smokers are stupid." While I don't agree that all smokers are stupid, I believe the act of smoking is stupid. With so much research regarding the toxic and deadly effects of smoking cigarettes, smoking really is a form of slow suicide. I find it ironic that insurance companies don't pay the families of suicide victims, yet they will pay the families of people who have died from smoking. Seems odd to me. If you're a smoker, respect yourself enough to stop. There are many effective programs and therapies. Discipline is the best one. No one else can quit for you. You are the only person who holds the cigarette to your mouth so you are the only one who can decide to treat your body with more respect by not lighting up.

If you don't have adequate respect for yourself or the discipline to quit, at the very least do not smoke around other people or hover at the doors of buildings so everyone else is forced to breathe the pollution you create. It unnerves and angers me when I see parents smoking around their children. I believe that parents who smoke around their children have no right to be parents. I think the Children's Aid Society should step in and protect children, who are even more vulnerable to the effects of second-hand smoke than adults, from the many deadly diseases they are inclined to suffer thanks to the neglect and abuse of their parents.

Toxic Street Drugs

Smoking marijuana is no better. Evidence links it to lung disease and cancer. The drug ecstasy has been linked to the destruction of brain cells, according to some research.[11] Cocaine, amphetamines, narcotics, and hallucinogens also put extreme stress on the body and create plentiful toxins in the body.

The High Cost of Beauty

The simple choice of which personal hygiene products such as soap, shampoo, hairspray, or deodorant you select can be affecting your health.

Unfortunately, our quest for beauty and attractiveness is often damaging to our bodies. Many toxins are found in cosmetics, skin-care products, and hair products. We slather on plentiful supplies of synthetic chemicals every time we wash, moisturize our skin, or apply cosmetics and hair products. It is ironic because the skin is the body's largest detoxification organ and not only are we hindering it from doing its important job, we are also adding more chemicals to our already overburdened bodies.

Most popular brands of cosmetics are loaded with artificial colours, synthetic fragrances, petroleum products, emulsifiers, preservatives, and solvents. Over 850 toxic chemicals are available for use in makeup. According to research by Dr. Patricia Fitzgerald, diethanolamine (DEA) and triethanolamine (TEA) are two particularly potent chemicals used in cosmetics. These chemicals combine with other chemicals to produce the carcinogens known as nitrosamines. The United States Food and Drug Administration found that 37 percent of the makeup tested contained nitrosamines.

The most common preservatives found in cosmetics and hygiene products are imidazolidinyl urea and diazolidinyl urea. Both chemicals are considered toxic and are well-researched causes of dermatitis (skin irritation). They also release formaldehyde at temperatures of 10 degrees C or higher. Numerous studies prove that formaldehyde is a carcinogen. That's right, it causes cancer.

Believe it or not, petroleum products are widely used in skin-care products and cosmetics as well. They can produce photosensitivity (promoting sensitivity to the sun) and interfere with the body's own natural moisturizing mechanism, leading to dry skin and chapping—the very problems these skin-care products are typically used to treat. One particular petroleum product, PVP/VA copolymer, is frequently used in hairsprays, wave sets for perms, and other cosmetics. This toxic substance may contribute to foreign particles in the lungs of a sensitive person.

Sodium lauryl sulfate, one of the synthetic substances that is used in shampoos and soaps for its foaming properties, causes eye irritations, skin rashes, hair loss, and allergic reactions. It is also a known mutagen, which means that it can cause changes in the information in your body's cellular genetic material, potentially leading to disease.

Stearalkonium chloride is another toxic chemical used in many hair conditioners and moisturizers. Originally developed by the fabric industry as a fabric softener, this toxic ingredient found its way into skin and hair products because it is much less expensive than proteins and natural ingredients. Unfortunately, this toxin also causes many allergic reactions.

As if that weren't enough, many synthetic colours are known cancer-causing agents. The synthetic colours used to make a cosmetic or hair dye "pretty" should be avoided at all costs. If personal-care products are labelled, these chemicals will appear as FD&C or D&C followed by a colour name and a number. For example, FD&C Red Number 6 or D&C Green Number 6. Many synthetic colours are cancer-causing agents. FD&C Red Number 2 was found to cause a statistically significant increase in a variety of cancers in female rats at the United States Federal Drug Administration's National Center for Toxicological Research. FD&C Blue Number 2 also produced malignant tumours in rats when it was injected under the skin. If a cosmetic contains synthetic colours, avoid purchasing it.

Synthetic fragrances used in cosmetics can also pose many health hazards. Consider that the single ingredient "fragrance" can have as many as four hundred ingredients, most of which are petrochemicals. Clinical observation by medical doctors has found that exposure to fragrances can damage the central nervous system and cause depression, hyperactivity, irritability, inability to cope, behavioural damages, headaches, dizziness, rashes, hyper-pigmentation, violent coughing, vomiting, coughing, and skin irritation.

Perfumes and colognes are the cosmetic equivalent of a wolf in sheep's clothing. At one time, perfumes and colognes were made from the pure essential oils found in flowers, tree resin, roots or bark, fruits, or other pure substances found in nature. According to the research of Julia Kendall (available at www.ehnca.org), the most common chemicals in perfumes are ethanol, benzaldehyde, benzyl acetate, a-pinene, acetone, benzyl alcohol, ethyl acetate, linalook, a-terpinene, methylene chloride, a-terpineol, camphor, and limonene. Smells beautiful, doesn't it? While some of these chemicals are harmless, most in this ingredient list cause irritability, mental vagueness, muscle pain, asthma, bloating, joint aches, sinus pain, fatigue, sore throat, eye irritation, gastrointestinal problems, laryngitis, headaches, dizziness, swollen lymph nodes, spikes in blood pressure, coughing, and burning or itching skin irritations. That perfume or cologne that you think makes you smell attractive is more likely damaging your health.

"A shocking 95 percent of the chemicals used in perfumes and colognes come from petroleum!"[12] I explain to my clients that many ingredients found in perfumes, colognes, and other fragrances are the by-products of the petroleum industry that cannot be used in vehicles or other industrial uses and so are sold as "beauty" products.

I challenge people to stay clear of all scented products for at least several months. I have yet to find a single person who thinks these products smell attractive after their sabbatical. Most often, people tell me that the perfume they loved so much smells more like Raid or Off. Because I have not used any scented products for many years, whenever I smell perfume or cologne, it really smells like someone sprayed their body with bug spray.

Some people incorrectly presume that only a toxic synthetic chemical will be potent enough to keep pests away. An Iowa State University research group showed that the essential oil found in the herb catnip is about ten times more effective than DEET in repelling mosquitoes in the laboratory. Also, an ingredient in neem seed oil (oil from the seeds of the neem tree are used for personal care products) has been found to be more effective than DEET by researchers at the Malaria Institute in India. Both the United States National Research Council and the *Journal of the American Mosquito Control Association* have confirmed this finding.[13]

Many people use baby products, thinking they are more natural and gentler for sensitive skin. Consider that high levels of 1,4 dioxane were recently found in samples of baby shampoo and conditioners. This chemical has been deemed an animal carcinogen and may pose a threat to humans as well.

Hair dyes usually contain coal tar colours that are linked to various forms of cancer, including non-Hodgkin's lymphoma. That doesn't mean you have to forfeit colouring your hair, rather, choose hennas and other natural products. The National Cancer Institute found that 20 percent of non-Hodgkin's lymphoma cases are related to synthetic colours in hair dye.[14]

Even most commercial brands of toothpaste are loaded with synthetic chemicals such as saccharin, FD&C Blue 1, and polysorbate 80, all of which are believed to be carcinogens. Fluoride is also suspected to increase cancer risk.

Feminine products such as tampons and sanitary pads are bleached, leaving a residue of dioxin, a known carcinogen that has been linked to immune disorders, endometriosis, and cancer of the reproductive system.

Ten of the Most Common Toxic Cosmetic Ingredients

1. Imidazolidinyl urea and diazolidinyl urea are the most commonly used preservatives after the parabens in the cosmetic industry. The American Academy of Dermatology has established that these two toxic ingredients are a primary cause of dermatitis (skin irritations). Two trade names for these chemicals are Germall II and Germall 115. Neither of the Germall chemicals is a good antifungal and must be combined with other preservatives. Germall 115 releases formaldehyde at just over 100 degrees F. Both chemicals are considered toxic.

2. Methyl, propyl, putyl, and ethyl paraben are used to inhibit microbial growth and to extend the shelf life of products. They are widely used even though they are known to be toxic and have caused many allergic reactions and skin rashes. They are highly toxic.

3. Petrolatum is mineral oil and jelly that causes a lot of problems when used on the skin. It can produce photosensitivity (promotes sun damage) and tends to interfere with the body's

own natural moisturizing mechanisms, leading to dry skin and chapping. Products containing petrolatum create the very conditions they claim to alleviate. Manufacturers use petrolatum because it is unbelievably cheap.

4. Propylene glycol is ideally a vegetable glycerin mixed with grain alcohol, both of which are natural. However, it usually appears as a synthetic petrochemical mix used as an emulsifier; it has been shown to cause allergic and toxic reactions.

5. PVP/VA copolymer is a petroleum-derived chemical used in hairsprays, wave sets, and other cosmetics. It is considered toxic, since particles may stay in the lungs of a sensitive person.

6. Sodium lauryl sulfate is a synthetic substance used in shampoos for its foam-building abilities. It causes eye irritations, skin rashes, hair loss, scalp scurf similar to dandruff, and allergic reactions. It is also frequently disguised in pseudo-natural cosmetics with the parenthetic explanation "comes from coconut."

7. Stearalkonium chloride is a chemical that causes allergic reactions and is used in hair conditioners and creams. Stearalkonium chloride was developed by the fabric industry as a fabric softener and is a lot cheaper and easier to use in hair-conditioning formulas than proteins or herbal ingredients but it is toxic.

8. The synthetic colours used to supposedly make a cosmetic "pretty" should be avoided at all costs, along with hair dyes. They will be labelled as FD&C or D&C followed by a colour and a number. Example: FD&C Red No. 6 or D&C Green No. 6. Synthetic colours are believed to be cancer-causing agents.

9. Synthetic fragrances used in cosmetics can have as many as four hundred ingredients. There is no way to know what the

chemicals are because the label will simply say "fragrance." Some of the many problems caused by these chemicals are headaches, dizziness, rash, hyperpigmentation, violent coughing, vomiting, and skin irritation. Advice: Don't buy a cosmetic that has the word *fragrance* on the ingredients label. If a cosmetic product doesn't list the ingredients, it usually contains synthetic fragrances and is best avoided.

10. Triethanolamine is frequently used in cosmetics to adjust the acid-alkaline balance (pH). It is also used with many fatty acids to convert acid to salt (stearate), which then becomes the base for a cleanser. TEA causes allergic reactions, including eye problems and dryness of hair and skin. It can also be toxic if absorbed into the body over a long period of time.

Source: Aubrey Hampton, *Natural Ingredients Dictionary Plus Ten Synthetic Cosmetic Ingredients to Avoid.*

HOME SWEET HOME

We often think of our home as our haven—the place we go to at the end of a long workday to relax, renew our energy, and simply be. While that is the case for some people, for others, home is the place where disease and illness begin. With every foam-filled attack on oven grease and grime, the scrubbing of every bathroom, and the spraying of air fresheners, another toxic chemical is released into the air, and into the bodies of the home's unsuspecting occupants.

Approximately fifty-four kilotons (equivalent of the weight of almost 137 fully-fuelled 747s) of all-purpose cleansers are used in Canadian homes every year. Their use affects human health and the quality of our fresh water and ground water, and increases health risks to wildlife, fish, and other aquatic life. The amount used by corporations and organizations is even higher.

In many studies, chemicals used in everyday household products have been found to cause health problems such as asthma and other respiratory ailments, birth defects, heart disease, and cancer. Of the more than eighty thousand synthetic chemicals widely used in our homes today, only 7 percent have been subjected to complete toxicity testing to determine the full extent of their health effects on people. And these tests have never determined the effects of household chemicals on children, pregnant women, elderly, or immune-compromised individuals.

In addition, there are no studies that examine the cumulative effects of chemicals on human health. For example, researchers have not explored the health implications of combining the many chemicals found in typical bathroom cleaning products.

A study conducted over fifteen years found that women who worked at home had a 54 percent higher death rate from cancer than women who had jobs outside of the home. The study concluded that the increased death rate was due to daily exposure to the hazardous chemicals found in ordinary household products, including so-called cleaning products.[15]

It is not difficult to understand the higher death rate when you consider the toxic effects of individual chemicals. For instance, chlorine, one of the most commonly used chemicals in cleaning products, is also one of the most toxic. It causes pain and inflammation of the mouth, throat, and stomach; erosion of mucous membranes; vomiting; circulatory collapse; confusion; delirium; coma; severe respiratory tract irritation; pulmonary edema; and skin eruptions. It has also been linked to high blood pressure, anemia, diabetes, heart disease, and gastrointestinal cancer. It is found in bleach, most scouring powders, disinfectants, and dishwashing detergents.

Ethanol, a grain derivative used in many household cleaners, causes central nervous system depression, anaesthesia, impaired motor coordination, double vision, vertigo, flushed face, nausea and vomiting, drowsiness, stupor, coma, dilated pupils, shock, hypo-thermia, and possibly death.

Two of the most common types of household products that contain ethanol are disinfectants and air fresheners. That's correct. Air fresheners contain harmful petroleum products. According to Michael Van Straten, British naturopath and osteopath and author of *Organic Living*, "Some air fresheners and fabric sprays reputedly work by blocking your sense of smell and attacking the tiny hairs in your nasal passages."

The United States National Public Health Service (a department of the Environmental Protection Agency) found that the chemical 1,4-dichlorobenzene (found in air fresheners) was found in the fat of 100 percent of people tested. This synthetic ingredient is irritating to the skin and mucous membranes.

What's more, the "fragrance" component in these products, as in cosmetics, can contain any of more than four hundred different ingredients, most of which are petrochemicals. Medical doctors have attributed central nervous system damage, depression, hyperactiv-ity, irritability, feelings of "inability to cope," and other behavioural effects to "fragrances."

Air fresheners are not the only toxins masquerading as safe home products. Don't forget all the hidden sources of toxic chemicals: bathroom cleaners, bleach, carpet shampoo, silver polish, window cleaner, oven cleaners, mould and mildew cleaners, scouring powders, laundry detergents, spot removers, drain cleaner, fabric softeners, dishwashing liquids, dishwasher detergents, floor cleaners, and furniture polish. These items are laden with artificial fragrances, formaldehyde, chlorine, petroleum distillates, perchloroethylene (known as "perc"), artificial colours, aerosol propellants, ammonia, cresol, ethanol, and many other chemicals.

Detergent, a seemingly harmless cleaning agent, is responsible for more household poisonings than any other substance. Exposure to this toxin can cause skin problems, asthma, flu-like symptoms, and other health problems.

Air fresheners, disinfectants, and mould and mildew cleaning products (among others) contain another harmful substance: formaldehyde. You learned a bit about formaldehyde earlier, when I discussed its use in cosmetics. In addition to being a suspected carcinogen, formaldehyde has been related to birth defects and genetic mutations in some studies. Symptoms from inhalation of formaldehyde vapours include cough, swelling of the throat, watery eyes, respiratory problems, throat irritation, headaches, rashes, tiredness, excessive thirst, nausea, nosebleeds, insomnia, disorientation, and asthma.

Conventional carpet shampoos contain toxic respiratory irritants that become airborne when the residue dries. Drain cleaners, oven cleaners, petroleum-based polyurethane floor and furniture finishes, and paint removers are extremely toxic and pollute the air.

In Canada, there are no laws that require all the ingredients of cleaning products to be listed on the label. So most products contain a blend of toxic chemicals that consumers inadvertently purchase and use regularly in their homes, believing they are safe.

The fumes of many cleaning products are actually quite noxious. Most people believe that hazardous chemicals are required to adequately disinfect their homes from any potential invading bacteria, viruses, moulds, fungi, or other pathogens. This is far from the truth and is having severe health ramifications. Keep in mind that most chemical cleaning products are relatively new—the chemical industry began in the 1940s. That is a relatively short time period in which to determine that they are safe for everyday exposure.

We also make the assumption that since our various levels of government allow these chemicals to be used then they must be safe. This is anything but true. The vast majority of chemicals that are currently used have never been studied for safety. Those that have been studied are rarely studied for long-term effects or multi-generational effects, nor have they been studied for their effects when combined with the many thousands of other chemicals human beings would normally come into contact with.

The regulatory process to create laws that govern the safety of products takes years to develop; new laws must be put through a consultation process (with the very industry that has a vested financial interest in making sure the products are allowed); they must be analyzed by lawyers, and then be published in government journals. What's more, there are no laws requiring manufacturers of household products to list the health effects of "normal" or long-term use of the product.

Clean and Healthy Home Quiz[16]

Take the following Clean and Healthy Home Quiz to see where you stand.

Give yourself the specified points for every "yes" answer. Score 0 for every "no" answer or if you use products purchased at natural food stores. However, if a product claims that it is "environmentally friendly," it may not necessarily be safe for your health. Score full points for these products.

1. Do you ever use drain or oven cleaners? Score 3 points.
2. Have you used carpet or upholstery shampoo in your current home or on existing furniture? Score 2 points for each type of product you have used (i.e., 2 points if you use carpet shampoo and 2 points if you also use upholstery shampoo).
3. Have you ever used professional carpet or upholstery cleaning services in your current home or on your existing furniture? Score 3 points for each type of service you have used in the last two years.
4. Do you use chemical bathroom cleaning products? Score 2 points.

5. Do you use bleach to clean your home or in your laundry? Score 2 points.

6. Do you use fabric softeners or dryer sheets? Score 3 points.

7. Do you ever use oven cleaners? Score 3 points.

8. Do you use dishwashing liquids or dishwasher detergents? Score 1 point for each type of product.

9. Do you use furniture polish? Score 1 point.

10. Do you use silver polish or stainless steel cleaner? Score 3 points.

11. Do you use mould and mildew cleaners? Score 2 points.

12. Do you use scouring powders or cream cleansers? Score 1 point.

13. Do you use window-cleaning products? Score 1 point.

14. Do you use floor cleaners? Score 1 point.

15. Do you use all-purpose cleaners? Score 2 points.

16. Do you use laundry detergents? Score 2 points.

17. Do you use spot removers for laundry? Score 2 points.

18. Do you dryclean your clothes? Score 3 points.

Scores: 27 to 43

You are exposing yourself and possibly your family to extremely high levels of toxic chemicals that are probably having effects on your health and energy levels. It is critical that you switch to natural products.

Scores: 11 to 26

You are breathing many toxic chemicals that are probably affecting your overall health and energy levels or will at some time in the future. Discontinue using many of the commercial brands of cleaning products in favour of natural ones.

Some of the Toxic Chemicals Found in Common Household Cleaning Products

Cleaning Product	Hazardous Substances
Air freshener	Naphthalene, phenol, cresol, ethanol, xylene, formaldehyde
All-purpose cleaner	Ammonia, detergents, artificial fragrances, aerosol propellants
Ammonia	Ammonia
Basin, tub, and tile cleaner	Detergents, artificial fragrances, aerosol propellants, chlorine
Bleach	Chlorine
Carpet shampoo	Perchloroethylene, naphthalene, ethanol, ammonia, detergents, artificial fragrance
Dishwashing detergent	Chlorine
Dishwashing liquid	Detergents, artificial fragrance, artificial colour, ammonia
Disinfectant	Cresol, phenol, ethanol, formaldehyde, ammonia, chlorine
Drain cleaner	Lye, ammonia, petroleum distillates

Fabric softener	Artificial fragrances
Floor/furniture polish	Phenol, nitrobenzene, acrylonitrile, ammonia, detergents, artificial fragrances, naphthalene, petroleum distillates, aerosol propellants
Laundry detergents	Detergents, bleaches, artificial fragrances
Mould and mildew cleaner	Phenol, kerosene, pentachlorophenol, formaldehyde
Oven cleaner	Lye, ammonia, aerosol propellants
Scouring powder (chlorinated)	Chlorine, detergents; talc may be contaminated with asbestos
Silver polish	Ammonia, petroleum distillates
Spot remover	Perchloroethylene
Window cleaner	Ammonia, artificial colours, aerosol propellants

Source: Debra Lynn Dadd, "Purify Your Home Without Poison," *Alternative Medicine,* April 2002, pp. 88–102.

The Top 20 Toxic Ingredients in Cleaning Products

Ingredient	Toxic Risks
Acrylonitrile	Suspected human carcinogen; can cause breathing difficulties, vomiting, diarrhea, nausea, weakness, headaches, and fatigue
Alkyl phenol ethoxylate (APE) surfactants (nonionic)	A large group of chemicals that are endocrine disruptors and have potential links in humans to tumours, cancers, and deformities

Aerosol propellants	Can cause heart problems, birth defects, lung cancer, headaches, nausea, dizziness, shortness of breath, eye and throat irritation, skin rashes, burns, lung inflammation, and liver damage
Ammonia (including ammonium chloride, quaternary compounds, benzalkonium chloride, etc.)	Can cause irritation of eyes and respiratory tract, conjunctivitis, laryngitis, tracheitis, pulmonary edema, pneumonitis and skin burns
Benzene	A carcinogen that can also cause drunk-like behaviour, light-headedness, disorientation, fatigue, and loss of appetite
Chlorine (including chlorine dioxide and sodium hypochlorite)	Can cause pain and inflammation of the mouth, throat, and stomach, erosion of mucous membranes, vomiting, circulatory collapse, confusion, delirium, coma, severe respiratory tract irritation, pulmonary edema, and skin eruptions. Has been linked to high blood pressure, anemia, diabetes, heart disease, and gastrointestinal cancer
Detergent	Responsible for more household poisonings than any other substance; exposure causes skin problems, flu-like and asthmatic conditions, severe eye damage, and severe upper digestive tract damage if ingested

Ethanol	Can cause central nervous system depression, anaesthesia, feelings of exhilaration, excessive talkativeness, impaired motor coordination, double vision, vertigo, flushed face, nausea and vomiting, drowsiness, stupor, coma, dilated pupils, shock, hypothermia, and possibly death
Formaldehyde	Suspected carcinogen; has been related to birth defects and genetic changes in bacteriological studies. Symptoms from inhalation of vapours include cough, swelling of the throat, watery eyes, respiratory problems, throat irritation, headaches, rashes, tiredness, excessive thirst, nausea, nosebleeds, insomnia, disorientation, and asthma
Kerosene	Can cause intoxication, ringing in the ears, burning sensation in chest, headaches, nausea, weakness, non-coordination, restlessness, confusion and disorientation, convulsions, coma, burning in the mouth, vomiting and diarrhea, drowsiness, rapid breathing, racing heart rate, fever, and death
Naphthalene	Suspected human carcinogen; can cause skin irritation, headaches, confusion, nausea and vomiting, excessive sweating, and urinary irritation. Exposure to sufficient quantity can cause death
Nitrobenzene	Can cause bluish skin, shallow breathing, vomiting, and death

Pentachlorophenol	Carcinogen; can also cause central nervous system depression, light-headedness, dizziness, sleepiness, nausea, tremor, loss of appetite, disorientation, and liver damage
Perchloroethylene	Inhaling fumes can cause cancer, liver damage, depression of the central nervous system, light-headedness, dizziness, sleepiness, nausea, loss of appetite, and disorientation
Petroleum distillates	A group of chemicals of varying toxicity that are made by distilling petroleum; they are suspected to be toxic to the kidneys, nervous system, respiratory system, and skin
Phenol	Suspected human carcinogen; causes skin eruptions and peeling, swelling, pimples, hives, burning, gangrene, numbness, vomiting, circulatory collapse, paralysis, convulsions, cold sweats, coma, and death
Sodium hydroxide (lye)	An extremely corrosive material that can eat right through skin; even a single dry crystal that falls on wet skin can cause damage. The exception is when lye is combined with fat in the making of soap. The chemical reaction neutralizes the sodium hydroxide, making the resulting soap safer to use

Sodium lauryl sulfate	Linked to harming children's eyes; contributes to hair loss and combines with DEA, MEA, and TEA (often found in the same product) to form nitrosamines, a carcinogen
Trichloroethylene	Suspected human carcinogen; also causes genetic mutations. Symptoms of exposure include gastrointestinal upsets, central nervous depression, heart and liver malfunctions, paralysis, nausea, dizziness, fatigue, and psychotic behaviour
Xylene	Can cause nausea, vomiting, excessive salivation, cough, hoarseness, feelings of euphoria, headaches, giddiness, vertigo, ringing in the ears, confusion, coma, and death

Source: Debra Lynn Dadd, "Purify Your Home Without Poison," *Alternative Medicine*, April 2002, pp. 88–102.

Other Toxins in Homes

Many homes built prior to 1970 were painted with lead-based paint. Lead can damage the heart, kidneys, and gastrointestinal tract, and being exposed to it can lead to brain damage.

In many studies second-hand smoke was found to be more damaging than smoking, and the many toxic chemicals found in cigarettes can remain in carpets, even after cleaning.

Most new carpeting off-gases formaldehyde and other respiratory irritants that can trigger asthma and allergies. Formaldehyde can also cause sneezing, eye irritation, and shortness of breath.

Toxic Lawn Care

If you use lawn and garden pesticides, herbicides, insecticides, or fungicides, you should know that many of these products approved for use on our lawns have been scientifically linked to Alzheimer's disease, cancer, and birth defects. I summarized the dangers of chemical use in gardens in my article in the *Ottawa Citizen*:

A new study on the illeffects of pesticides pops up faster than you can say, "DDT." The University of Rochester School of Medicine and Dentistry conducted a study of a common herbicide, paraquat, and fungicide, maneb. Mice that were subjected to these chemicals developed the same pattern of brain damage seen in Parkinson's disease. Parkinson's is a progressive brain illness that initiates tremors and eventually paralysis. It is the illness that actor Michael J. Fox, boxer Muhammad Ali, and Pope John Paul II suffer from.

A study by the Canadian Institute of Child Health found that even small amounts of chemicals like pesticides have negative effects on children's development.

In other studies, breast cancer has been linked to pesticide and fertilizer use. The highest incidence of breast cancer in the United States was found in the areas of Long Island, New York, that were heavily sprayed with DDT. Female workers who have been exposed to dioxin have higher rates of breast cancer than the general public.

Another study of 229 New York women found that women who developed breast cancer had higher levels of PCBs, DDEs, and other pesticides in their fat stores than women who did not develop the disease.

And, the evidence is not limited to pesticides. Fertilizer is not the harmless, lawn supportive stuff it appears to be either. A recent study by the Public Interest Research Groups (PIRG) indicates that "fertilizers made from industrial wastes are contaminating farms, gardens, and lawns, and eventually food and people, with toxic metals (twenty-two were found, including endocrine disruptors arsenic and lead) at levels higher than allowed in public landfills.

Every now and then a study is unveiled that indicates pesticides are not causing damage. Most of them do not take into consideration long-term exposure, the cumulative effect of pesticides and other chemicals our bodies are exposed to throughout our lifetimes, and the simple fact is there are people who have compromised immune systems, and of course, children whose bodies are developing. All these people are more susceptible to the effects of pesticides and other "lawn-care" chemicals than the mythical "average adult."[17]

INDUSTRIAL AIRBORNE CHEMICALS

Synthetic chemicals contaminate every part of the planet, even the most isolated and remote areas.

Of the more than eighty thousand synthetic chemicals widely used today, only 7 percent have been subjected to complete toxicity testing to determine the full extent of their health effects on people. These tests have not been specific enough to determine their effects on the growing bodies of children, immune-compromised individuals, or seniors, their cumulative effects, or the effects of combining them.

Industrial chemicals find their way into the human body through the air we breathe, the water we bathe in, and soil in which our food is grown. According to Dr. Patricia Fitzgerald, "Levels of toxicity in the human body, as well as on the planet, have been higher in the past twenty years than in the entire history of the world."[18]

In his book, *Healing the Planet One Patient at a Time*, Dr. Jozef Krop's research indicates that breast milk in women in Western countries is so seriously contaminated that it would not pass American Food and Drug Administration standards if it were a packaged product. He adds, "In the Eastern seaboard and southwestern United

States (the most highly industrialized parts), mothers are not recommended to breastfeed past six months, as the baby by then already has the maximum lifetime amounts of carcinogens in its cells."

Dr. Krop also cites a recent report that indicated toxic air triggers one thousand premature deaths and five thousand hospitalizations per year in Toronto alone. Poor air quality is linked to heart attacks, cardiovascular disease, asthma, and lung cancer, and it can be a factor in many other illnesses. According to the American Cancer Society, environmental toxins might account for as many as three-quarters of all cancers.[19]

Dr. Fitzgerald states: "In 1992 alone, the Environmental Protection Agency received official notice from companies that 273 million pounds of toxic waste had been dumped into surface water. We can only wonder how much additional discharge into our waters went unreported. Another 338 million pounds of toxic waste were deposited on land that year, and 726 million pounds illegally injected underground."[20]

She continues, "A 1999 government study on air pollution in Los Angeles found the risk of cancer in that city to be 426 TIMES greater than health standards established by the 1990 Federal Clean Air Act."[21] According to her research, "The primary pollution source in L.A. is motor vehicles, with diesel exhaust from trucks and buses having a significant share of the detrimental impact."[22]

According to Dr. Krop, some estimates suggest that the average person breathes two tablespoons of assorted particles into his or her lungs every day. In more polluted city centres or areas near industrial sites, that amount can be significantly higher.

In Canada, people often rely on the Air Quality Index (AQI) reported by Environment Canada to determine the safety of the air they breathe. With thousands of chemicals being emitted into the air, you may be alarmed to find that this index provides a reading on only six common city air pollutants to determine air quality.

They are:
- carbon monoxide
- nitrogen dioxide
- ozone
- suspended particles,
- total reduced sulphur
- sulphur dioxide.[23]

KEEP IT MOVING

Exercise or, more aptly, lack of exercise also plays a tremendous role in the way toxins affect the body. Exercise helps the body's cells absorb greater volumes of oxygen, enabling the cells to become purer; it also helps the lymphatic and circulatory systems remove damaging toxins from your tissues and blood. By sweating, you better enable your body to eliminate toxins through your skin. So if you are in the group of 20 to 25 percent of people who do not exercise, you are allowing toxins to build up in your body. If you are like the additional 33 percent of people, you probably are not moving enough to reap any health benefits of exercise.[24]

There are many benefits of exercising:
- increases energy
- reduces stress
- burns fat
- speeds metabolism
- builds bone mass
- increases oxygen supply to the tissues and organs
- builds muscle
- improves posture
- increases lung capacity and strength
- increases flexibility
- strengthens joints
- balances the spine and hips

- increases bodily awareness
- balances the brain
- calms the mind
- leads to greater relaxation
- increases self-confidence
- aids weight loss or gain (as needed).

On the flip side, if you're not exercising adequately, you may be tired, stressed, and overweight and have a slow metabolism or low bone mass. You may have inadequate oxygen for healthy tissues and organs, or worse, you may already have diseased tissues and organs. You may have poor muscle tone and posture, inadequate lung capacity and strength, rigid joints, imbalanced spine and hips, poor bodily awareness, or imbalanced left and right hemispheres of your brain. You may have difficulty relaxing and suffer from inadequate self-confidence.

If you're like most people you're probably saying, "Yeah, yeah, I know exercise is good for me, but I hate the stuff." Like it or not, exercise is a component of *The 4-Week Ultimate Body Detox Plan.* You may be surprised to learn that it incorporates exercise that doesn't have to be difficult or cumbersome. On the contrary, it will be fun and easier than you think. One of the main types of exercise that is included in the program is walking.

Walking is fabulous. It reduces the risk of cancer, heart disease, and stroke; has a very low injury risk level; decreases the risk of diabetes by improving your body's ability to use insulin; helps prevent osteoporosis by strengthening your bones; can help you lose weight, sleep better, reduce stress and depression, ease PMS and menopausal symptoms, and much more. A recent study found that walking lowers cholesterol levels.[25] Another study conducted by the Appalachian State University found that women who walked for forty-five minutes per day recovered twice as fast from colds as women who did not exercise.[26] A study at a medical centre in Salt Lake City found that walking after eating moved food through the stomach more quickly, helping to relieve minor indigestion.[27] The *Berkeley Wellness Letter* has cited walking as the perfect exercise for promoting a healthy back.

Researchers at the Center for Health and Fitness at the University of Massachusetts found that people who took a brisk forty-minute walk felt a 14 percent drop in anxiety levels.[28]

As if all of that were not enough, walking also contributes to a healthy relationship. A study at the Exercise, Physiology and Human Performance Laboratory at the University of California at San Diego found that healthy men aged thirty-five to sixty-five who started a regular exercise program hugged and kissed their wives more often and had more sexual intercourse and more orgasms than those who did not exercise. Dare I add that regular exercise might have added to their endurance in the bedroom?

Walking also lowers blood pressure, reduces the risk of colon cancer, boosts the immune system, and stimulates the lymphatic system.[29] You may not be surprised to learn that I will be asking you to walk throughout *The 4-Week Ultimate Body Detox Plan*. Yes, there are other programs out there that will tell you that exercise is not really necessary for results. I don't want to be rude, but they are lying to you, or at least appeasing you. That's what most people want to hear. But we all know in our hearts and minds that exercise *is* necessary. Only you can get those limbs moving.

LIVING IN A TOXIC WORLD

What happens to all these toxins once they enter the body? The intestines eliminate some waste products through bowel movements; the liver filters other toxins, as do the kidneys. Additional toxins are excreted through the skin. The lungs remove some toxins, while the lymphatic system sweeps out others. The bloodstream tackles some toxins, and the colon eliminates others. But often the body simply cannot keep up with the vast amount of toxins we are exposed to. What happens then? Well, the detoxification organs work as hard as they are able. Some will overwork as long as they can but eventually they become sluggish and ineffective at doing their jobs.

Dr. Paula Baillie-Hamilton, author of *The Body Restoration Plan*, says, "In effect, most of the chemicals that we cannot eliminate end up being stored in our adipose tissue (body fat) due to their high fat solubility. Contrary to popular belief, however, once in the fat stores they are not out of harm's way, because once there they set to work damaging our fat metabolism."[30]

That's right: toxins can make you fat. They can also make it more difficult to lose weight. But that's not all. They are often implicated in many other diseases and disorders.

The Toxin-Disease Connection

I believe that toxins are implicated in almost every disease or disorder that ails humankind, including autoimmune diseases such as arthritis, lupus, multiple sclerosis, chronic fatigue syndrome, and fibromyalgia; hormonal imbalances such as premenstrual syndrome, menopausal symptoms, and others; psychological disturbances such as depression, bipolar syndrome, schizophrenia, mood swings, and irritability; obesity; digestive disorders; metabolic disorders; cancer; and brain diseases such as Alzheimer's and Parkinson's.

We have bought in to the notion that our parents passed down bad genes and those genes are the main culprit in disease. We believe we are victims of circumstance. Genes may be a factor, but usually they play a minimal role.

Or perhaps we blame a microscopic organism: a virus, bacteria, or fungus that we cannot even see, yet it has this immense power over our bodies. Pathogens such as viruses and bacteria may play a small role in illness but a normal healthy immune system should be able to keep them in check.

Or maybe we blame aging for what ails us. After all, the average elderly person is hardly the picture of health. Yet there are aged people who defy this notion entirely. I just saw photographs in a health magazine of an eighty-year-old woman and Pilates instructor who is the picture of physical fitness as she contorts her body into positions most twenty-year-olds would balk at.

Genes, pathogens, and aging are factors in our health but toxins play a much greater role. If toxins build up faster than they can be removed, disease results—not necessarily immediately but it *is* the result. Sometimes we feel fatigued, lethargic, weak, or headachy. Sometimes we pack on the pounds or suffer from aches and pains. These symptoms are the result of toxic overload—too many toxins building up and not enough being eliminated.

As desperate as the situation sounds, it is not... if we take measures to eliminate the vast quantity of harmful toxins we expose ourselves to. As you will see in the following chapters, you do not need to be a helpless victim or an ignorant bystander while your body struggles. You will learn how you can reduce your exposure to toxins and improve your body's capacity to eliminate them.

In this chapter you learned
+ What you think about all day long has substantial effects on creating a healthy or unhealthy body
+ Unmanaged stress creates toxins in your body
+ There are thousands of toxic chemicals in cigarette smoke
+ There are many sources of air pollution and that air quality indexes do not adequately inform us about many of these pollutants
+ Many household cleaning products are not as safe as you may think
+ Chemicals in hair- and body-care products and cosmetics are

absorbed through your skin, adding further burden to your body's detoxification organs.

References

1. Richard Gerber, *Vibrational Medicine for the 21st Century* (New York: HarperCollins Publishers, Inc., 2000), p. 101.

2. Gerber, *Vibrational Medicine for the 21st Century*, p. 107.

3. Michelle Cook, "Harness the Power of Love," *Ottawa Citizen*, February 14, 2001.

4. Jacqueline Krohn and Frances Taylor,. *Natural Detoxification: A Practical Encyclopedia* (Port Roberts, WA: Hartley & Marks Publishers, Inc., 2000).

5. "Detoxification." Informational Brochure. Advanced Nutrition Publications, Inc., 1994.

6. David E. Root and Joan Anderson, "Reducing Toxic Body Burdens Advancing in Innovative Technique," *Occupational Health and Safety News Digest* 2, April 1986.

7. Root and Anderson, "Reducing Toxic Body Burdens Advancing in Innovative Technique."

8. Maya Muir, "Ridding the Body of Toxic Chemicals: Detoxification Protocols," *Alternative & Complementary Therapies*, August 1998.

9. Patricia Fitzgerald, *The Detox Solution* (Santa Monica, CA: Illumination Press, 2001), p. 89.

10. Fitzgerald, *The Detox Solution*, p. 89.

11. Fitzgerald, *The Detox Solution*, p. 91.

12. Fitzgerald, *The Detox Solution*, p. 87.

13. Paul Henderson, "Neem and Catnip Oil Repels Mosquitoes Best," *Vitality Magazine*.

14. Fitzgerald, *The Detox Solution*, p. 87.

15. Dadd, Debra Lynn. "Purify Your Home Without Poison." *Alternative Medicine* magazine. Issue No. 47, April 2002.

16. Michelle Schoffro Cook , "Home Sweet Home," *Health 'N' Vitality*, [**date or volume and issue number?**] pp. 28–29.

17. Michelle Cook, "Is Your Lawn Worth Your Health?" *Ottawa Citizen*, June 5, 2001.

18. Fitzgerald, *The Detox Solution*, p. 40.

19. Fitzgerald, *The Detox Solution*, p. 27.

20. Fitzgerald, *The Detox Solution*, p. 41.

21. Fitzgerald, *The Detox Solution*, p. 45.

22. Fitzgerald, *The Detox Solution*, p. 45.

23. Jozef J. Krop, *Healing the Planet One Patient at a Time* (Alton, ON: KOS Publishing, Inc., 2002), p. 81.

24. Fitzgerald, *The Detox Solution*, p. 91.

25. Harvey Diamond, *The Fit for Life Solution* (St. Paul, MN: Dragon Door Publications, Inc., 2002), p. 164.

26. Diamond, *The Fit for Life Solution*, p. 164.

27. Diamond, *The Fit for Life Solution*, p. 164.

28. Diamond, *The Fit for Life Solution*, p. 164.

29. Diamond, *The Fit for Life Solution*, p. 164.

30. Paula Baillie-Hamilton, *The Body Restoration Plan* (New York, NY: Avery, 2003), p. 22.

CHAPTER 4

The Gentle Detox Solution

*Each one of the substances of a man's diet acts upon his body and
changes it in some way, and upon these changes, his whole life
depends, whether he be in health, in sickness, or convalescent.*
Hippocrates

In this chapter you will learn
- How detoxification helps create greater energy, balance weight,
  eliminate negative symptoms, reduce cellulite, and much more
- About the major detoxification organs and how they help your
  body eliminate toxins and toxic buildup
- What to expect while detoxifying
- How to start eliminating toxins from your environment by
  choosing healthier cleaning and personal-care products
- Why *The 4-Week Ultimate Body Detox Plan* is uniquely suited
  to reduce or eliminate the side effects commonly associated
  with detoxifying as well as provide a thorough cleansing to *all*
  your body's detox organs

Diana is like many women: she unknowingly exposes herself to more toxins than she could ever imagine. She rises early to begin her day with her morning shower, which exposes her to chlorine and other water contaminants. She lathers her body with a liquid soap that smells and looks pretty (and is full of colours, fragrances, sudsing agents, and other chemicals), washes and conditions her hair with shampoo and conditioner that expose her to more chemicals. She slathers on creams and lotions full of synthetic chemicals that will be absorbed by her skin—her body's largest detoxification organ. She uses deodorant containing the heavy metal aluminum among other toxic substances. Then she spritzes herself with perfume that is loaded with harmful ingredients that also are absorbed through her skin and that she inhales all day long. After blow-drying her hair, she sprays it with chemical-laden hairspray that exposes her skin and lungs to further toxins. Diana loves wearing beautiful clothes but they secretly hide harmful laundry soaps, fabric softeners, or dry-cleaning chemicals.

She takes pride in what she refers to as her "mostly healthy eating habits" and encourages her teenage children to eat similarly. She eats a whole-grain cereal with milk or whole-wheat toast every morning. The cereal she consumes contains preservatives and plentiful amounts of sugars disguised by their names. The milk contains growth hormones, synthetic estrogen, antibiotics, and other medications used in the raising of dairy cows. She chugs back a glass of orange juice that is also laden with sugar and still contains residue of the pesticides, herbicides, fungicides, fertilizers, and other chemicals used to grow the oranges. She grabs an apple for the drive to work—"After all, an apple a day keeps the doctor away," she tells herself.

On the drive to work she breathes exhaust fumes containing many harmful toxins found in petrochemicals, alongside other air pollutants from industrial plants, cigarette smoke, and thousands of chemicals found in air pollution. Arriving at her office job, she inhales formaldehyde from the new desks, chairs, and other office furniture.

The building itself is only a year old and is still giving off the gas of many chemicals used in the manufacture of the synthetic materials. She unknowingly inhales these toxins with every breath. She rushes off to the laser printer to grab the document she has been working on and then makes numerous copies on the photocopier, the whole time breathing additional chemicals from the toner.

Janice, her friend and co-worker, passes her in the hall wearing a lovely new perfume that Diana immediately notices and admires (breathing further synthetic chemicals). But Diana still catches the odour of cigarette smoke that the perfume was intended to mask.

On her drive home after work, she sighs with fatigue, then notices the flashing neon of fast-food row. She internally debates whether she really has enough energy to make dinner tonight and finally decides to stop for food, after all, "that fried chicken really isn't so bad occasionally, is it?" Along with the chicken, she grabs the bag of buns and four colas and heads for home. The kids will be nicely surprised. Diana would be surprised too if she saw the list of synthetic flavours, colours, dough conditioners, sugar and synthetic sweeteners, hormones, and other chemicals making up this "meal."

After dinner she can barely scrape together enough energy to do some laundry (with chemical-laden soap and fabric-softener sheets). "It's a good thing I picked up dinner tonight so I have enough energy to do a bit of housekeeping—well, a load or two of laundry," she tells herself reassuringly, then heads for bed.

The number of toxic chemical exposures Diana encountered during her day is in the thousands. This is true for most people.

In Chapters 2 and 3 you learned about the myriad toxins present in our foods, homes, and all around us. The number of toxins to which we are regularly exposed sounds overwhelming, and our bodies may be feeling the same way. However, some minor changes to your daily routine and a little awareness about positive choices you can make will result in substantially fewer toxins for your body to cope with. As well, you are about to learn a powerful detoxification method that will help you feel great every day while allowing your body to efficiently eliminate toxins and improve the functioning of your detox organs.

Nature created our bodies to have innate mechanisms to prevent an overflow of toxins. Although we have overwhelmed these systems, we can help to restore them to optimal functioning. Enter *The 4-Week Ultimate Body Detox Plan*. After years of trying virtually every form of cleansing, I found that some worked while others did not. I found that almost every cleansing method involved negative symptoms and cleansing reactions. The authors of these plans said that these symptoms were a necessary evil: "no pain, no gain."

I tried liver detoxes, gallbladder flushes, colon cleanses, toning and purifying herbs. I drank nothing but lemon juice in water with maple syrup for one program; during another I ate only apples for days; still another program had me popping over sixty nutritional supplements. I sickened of apples, grapefruit, and lemon juice. I tired of pill-popping. I thought only of the gourmet and decadent foods I would eat at the end of these harsh programs. I felt a bit like a character in Clement Clarke Moore's *Twas the Night Before Christmas*—I was the one with visions of sugarplums dancing in my head. I also had visions of chocolate, pasta, and pie.

At the end of most programs, I felt modestly improved or unchanged. On some cleansing programs, I felt worse than when I started. On one program, my body actually swelled. I felt like a balloon on a helium machine. My legs became so bloated I could barely put weight on them without discomfort. I looked and felt terrible. One thing became abundantly clear to me: there had to be a more effective and less painful way to cleanse one's body.

My quest for the ultimate detoxification program resulted in *The 4-Week Ultimate Body Detox Plan*. I discovered that the results of other programs would always be minimal because they targeted one or two detoxification organs in the body—usually the liver or the colon. So I devised a program that targeted the whole digestive tract, the liver and gallbladder, the skin, the kidneys and urinary tract, fatty deposits in the body, the lymphatic system, and the bloodstream and cardiovascular system. Now I was getting somewhere. I started to feel immensely better than before.

But I still experienced some side effects of cleansing. I discovered that whether you target one or all of the cleansing mechanisms in the body, it is imperative that you cleanse *in the right order*. I tested my theory, and the results were substantially improved. Although you may experience some minor symptoms of cleansing (depending on how toxic your body is), these symptoms will be greatly reduced. You may experience no symptoms at all. By following *The 4-Week Ultimate Body Detox Plan*, you will experience greater energy, less pain, and improved mental clarity. You may even experience freedom from the nagging symptoms of disease that have plagued you for years.

DETOXIFICATION 101

Dr. Elson Haas, at the Preventive Medical Center of Marin in San Rafael, California, defines a toxin as "any substance that creates irritating and/or harmful effects in the body, undermining our health or stressing our biochemical or organ functions." And, as you learned earlier, detoxification is the process of cleansing the body of these harmful substances, thereby restoring the body's natural healing ability. There are many different types of detoxification processes, ranging from water fasts to programs that have minor dietary restrictions. Some programs use herbs, while others use foods. Some cleansing plans incorporate exercise while others do not.

Like many people, you may be looking for the "miracle pill" or the "magic program" that requires little or no effort on your part.

I can guarantee that pills or programs that prevent your participation in the approach taken will yield few, if any, results. Their lists of claims make up for the lack of effort expected from you, and surprise: they simply do not work!

During *The 4-Week Ultimate Body Detox Plan*, you will be an active participant in your own life. While this may sound like an obvious statement, it is actually rare in the world of medicine and healing. You will eat the foods, drink the teas, and perform the exercises. What's more, you will feel empowered that you are restoring your body to its optimum functioning. You will feel great, knowing that *you* are creating the sense of well-being that comes from following this program. You will have taken charge of your life and you will thank yourself upon completion. If you are like most people who follow this program, you will savour the delicious foods, you will enjoy the simple, at-home therapies, and you will appreciate the stress-relieving techniques.

The 4-Week Ultimate Body Detox Plan incorporates herbs, foods, juices, aromatherapy, exercise, breathing techniques, and many other enjoyable therapies. Most importantly, you will give your body a break from dietary and lifestyle habits that may be wreaking havoc on your health.

Detoxification is often referred to as fasting. I distinguish between the two concepts. Traditionally, fasting has meant water fasts, whereas detoxification can be any number of different types of programs, ranging from grapefruit or apple diets, to juice fasts, to ones that incorporate foods as well. I am not a fan of water fasts because I think they have the potential to be dangerous, particularly in people who have pre-existing health concerns. Even when relieved of the burden of excess food the body, still has specific nutritional requirements that cannot be met by water alone. Your brain has high fuel requirements, particularly for natural sugars. If your body is not supplied with this fuel, it will break down muscle tissue by day two of the fast or it will enter a process known as ketosis.

Ketosis is a process by which your liver converts stored fat and other nonessential tissue into substances called ketones, which can then be used by the brain, muscles, and heart as energy. This is the process that high-protein, low-carb diet proponents encourage to achieve fat-burning. It works to eliminate excess weight; however, over long periods of time, ketosis can be dangerous. Your body thinks it is starving.

As you will learn later in this chapter, many nutrients are required for your body to be able to conduct the many processes of detoxification. Without any of them, toxins will build up faster than they can be eliminated.

The 4-Week Ultimate Body Detox Plan does not incorporate water fasts. You will never starve on this plan. Neither will you eat only apples for days or skip meals. Instead, you will enjoy the foods and beverages you eat and drink so much that you will forget you are following a detoxification program.

Does Detoxification Really Work?

While many misinformed or, more accurately, uninformed journalists and health professionals may tell you otherwise, the resounding answer is *yes*. The approach taken in *The 4-Week Ultimate Body Detox Plan* helped give me my life back. Many of my clients with whom I use detoxification therapy share the same feeling. Ronnie stopped suffering from chronic back pain that she had endured for over six years within one month; Norm had severe fibromyalgia that relented within one month; Jane needed more extensive detoxification but was able to stop using depression medication after several months of cleansing, and her moods have been substantially improved; Connie's debilitating fibromyalgia totally subsided within one month; Kirk is free from seasonal allergies and sinus problems that had bothered him most of his life after just one month of cleansing; and Darla's high blood pressure normalized in two months. Others who have tried it have experienced weight loss, increased energy, the easing or elimination of arthritic symptoms, and much more. Research shows that detoxification works. Various detoxification approaches were used in the studies that follow, but all had statistically significant results.

In one study, conducted at the Center for Conservative Therapy in Penngrove, California, 174 patients who were suffering from hypertension participated in an eleven-day fast. By the end of the study, 90 percent of the participants achieved a blood pressure reading of 140/90—substantially improved over their starting blood pressure. The people who had the worst hypertension at the beginning of the study had the most significant improvement in blood pressure. Many were able to eliminate their blood pressure medication. Forty-two of the patients were able to maintain the improvements after the study concluded.[1]

In a Norwegian study, researchers found that fasting may help alleviate the symptoms of rheumatoid arthritis. Twenty-seven arthritic patients adhered to a four-week detoxification program followed by strict vegetarian diets. After one year, the patients reported significantly less pain, stiffness, and swelling, as well increased strength and better health.[2]

Laboratory experiments also found that short-term detoxification may even help you live longer.[3]

During one study, researchers at Kyushu University in Fukuoka, Japan, found that mice that fasted for four consecutive days every two weeks had a significantly longer lifespan than the mice that ate a typical diet.[4]

The National Institute on Aging found that detoxification increases a person's lifespan as well as or better than caloric restriction.[5]

Still more research has shown that periodically fasting for short periods of time lowers LDL (the "bad") cholesterol, boosts insulin sensitivity, stimulates the release of growth hormones, reduces the rate of viral infections, helps protect the brain from excitotoxins (a category of synthetic food ingredients, characterized by a dangerous combination of amino acids that overstimulate the nervous system—examples of excitotoxins includ MSG and aspartame), and improves the quality of sleep, concentration, vigour, and emotional balance.[6]

These are just a handful of the studies that show detoxification works. More studies are needed to prove the beneficial effects of detoxification, but I am convinced more time and money will result in additional studies that show how promising detoxification can be. Those of us who actually try it, don't need the studies to confirm the difference in how we feel.

With *The 4-Week Ultimate Body Detox Plan*, the results of cleansing all your body's detoxification organs will positively surprise you.

THE DETOXIFICATION ORGANS

There are many organs in your body whose primary function is to eliminate waste products: either those that are created internally like stress hormones (endotoxins) or those that come from our food, air, pharmaceuticals, lifestyle habits, and environment (exotoxins). Your body has numerous detoxification systems to deal with different types of toxins. These include:

- the digestive system, particularly the intestines, liver, and gallbladder
- the kidneys and urinary tract
- the lymphatic system
- the skin
- the lungs and respiratory system
- the bloodstream and cardiovascular system
- fatty deposits (while not officially a detox system, this is a mechanism your body uses when too many toxins threaten to overload the other systems)

Most of these systems have numerous organs that they depend on to help the whole system function smoothly.

A Brief Tour of the Digestive System

The digestive system comprises many organs, but the main ones we will be dealing with are the stomach, small intestine, large intestine (also known as the colon), liver, and gallbladder. Although teeth are not frequently included in texts about the digestive system, I am also including them, as well as salivary glands and the mouth. When you eat food, digestion begins immediately. Your teeth grind food into smaller particles that can be handled by the other digestive organs, and the salivary glands secrete digestive juices full of substances called enzymes. These enzymes break down foods such as starches and sugars.

Mom was right when she told you to chew your food well. If you don't, your body misses one whole step of digestion. This process is not performed by another part of the digestive tract. After you swallow, the food passes through the esophagus down into the stomach. In the stomach, secreted hydrochloric acid is released to break down protein foods.

Intestinal Tract

The food then passes into the small intestines, where nutrients and toxins are absorbed by the intestinal wall and passed into the bloodstream. Without regular bowel movements (after every meal), toxic waste starts to accumulate on the walls of the bowels and is absorbed into the blood. It may even prevent nutrients from being absorbed.

The liver produces a green-coloured substance called bile and sends it to the gallbladder for storage and secretion as necessary. The gallbladder secretes bile to help break down fat and stimulate contractions of the intestines to push waste matter out of your bowels. Then the remaining waste products are pushed down into the large intestine. The digestive tract is a tube that runs approximately thirty-five feet through your body. In addition to digesting food, it absorbs nutrients and eliminates remaining waste products. One hundred times greater than the area of your skin,[7] it contains massive numbers of microorganisms to assist with these functions. Actually, there are more microorganisms found in your digestive tract than there are cells in your body.[8]

It is believed that many of these organisms make essential nutrients that our bodies need to live and that are absorbed into the bloodstream through the intestinal walls. However, some of these organisms can become overgrown, primarily due to our unhealthy lifestyles, which are loaded with sugar, harmful fats, synthetic chemicals, and stress hormones; other factors play a role, too. When these organisms become overgrown, some of them can create harmful toxins that also pass through the walls of the intestines.

When the intestines are not kept "flushed" of toxic residue and buildup, this fecal matter along with the accompanying toxins and harmful bacteria can be re-absorbed into the bloodstream, where it can travel throughout the body. This is because vitamins and minerals that are extracted from food are absorbed into the bloodstream through the walls of the intestines. If debris is backed up in the intestines, it is absorbed into the bloodstream instead of the nutrients. Not only does your body become self-intoxicating, it cannot adequately take up the nutrients it needs for maintaining its health.

Toxic buildup in the intestines can result in virtually any health problem by simply allowing toxins to travel throughout the body via the bloodstream and by preventing nutrients from being absorbed from the food you eat *and the supplements you take.* That's right. If your intestines are backed up, no amount of pill-popping is going to mean good health. You can pop all the calcium or vitamin C, or any other vitamin or mineral supplement, you want but your body will not be able to absorb it.

The Liver and Gallbladder

The liver is a relatively large organ that sits beneath the rib cage on the right side of the body. With over five hundred functions, it has more jobs than any other organ in the body. It is critical to good health that the liver function up to par. It has the task of metabolizing fats, carbohydrates, and proteins. It also metabolizes hormones, foreign chemicals, and wastes that are created within your body as a by-product of day-to-day living and all the functions that entails—day-to-day living results in the creation of many by-products. It is responsible for forming bile and lymph, both of which will be discussed in a moment. The liver produces blood-clotting factors and helps with the assimilation and storage of fat-soluble vitamins. In addition to these vitamins, the liver stores carbohydrates and minerals. This powerhouse organ also helps to regulate blood sugar levels by storing excess blood sugar as a substance called glycogen, which can be released and converted into glucose (sugar) for energy when your body needs it.

The gallbladder is a small organ that looks like a little bag tucked under the liver. Connected to the liver in an area between the stomach and the intestines, the gallbladder collects bile from the liver and pumps it into the intestines as needed. Bile is a greenish-yellow liquid that assists with the removal of waste products from the intestines and helps break down fat.

The Kidneys and Urinary Tract

The kidneys are two small organs in the abdominal area that have several main functions: they strive to maintain balance in your body, particularly fluid and sodium balances; excrete toxins in urine; and regulate blood pressure through hormone production. Our main concern is with the first two functions. However, the kidneys secrete a hormone that increases blood pressure to allow sufficient pressure in the blood entering the kidneys, thereby enabling them to adequately perform their filtering functions. By lessening your toxic load, you may notice that your blood pressure normalizes as well.

The kidneys allow most substances to enter the urine, then they filter it and reabsorb the many compounds that the body needs. Some of these substances include glucose (simple sugars that your body needs to function), amino acids, and minerals that were circulating unabsorbed in the bloodstream.

Many of the toxins that are created as by-products of normal metabolic functions in the body are excreted in the urine, via the kidneys.

Kidneys also regulate the amount of fluid in your body: if you drink more, you urinate more, and vice versa. This prevents your body from becoming dehydrated or overhydrated. Your kidneys also monitor salt levels. Most people consume far more of the mineral sodium than they need so this puts a fair amount of stress on the kidneys.

According to some research, sodium was scarce in Stone Age times, yet the mineral potassium was found in abundance in all the plant foods our ancestors ate. In response, the kidneys developed a mechanism to more readily store sodium and excrete potassium, the opposite of what is needed based on our modern diet. This excess sodium strains your kidneys and makes them work harder to maintain a proper mineral balance in your body. Detoxifying your diet of excess sodium, as we will do in *The 4-Week Ultimate Body Detox Plan*, will allow your kidneys to focus their energy on the important task of eliminating toxins from your body.

The kidneys also attempt to maintain the acid/alkaline balance in your body. This is an immensely difficult task because the average North American person's diet is largely acidic. The high level of acidity means that your kidneys will have to work harder to perform their jobs and may eventually become sluggish from overwork.

All the kidney's jobs require adequate fluid intake. If you do not drink enough water, your kidneys simply cannot function up to par, and your body's cells will become dehydrated, making virtually every function in your body less efficient. Most people do not drink enough water to adequately bathe the cells in fluid to enable them to function properly. That lack spells trouble if it is not rectified.

THE SKIN YOU'RE IN

Skin is the body's largest organ. It shields our bodies from the elements around us (sometimes taking a beating in the process), assists with detoxification, and protects our tissues and organs from damage. It is also a reflection of the condition of our bodies at a deeper level. Skin reflects our inner health. It may show up toxic overload, stress, hormonal imbalances, and nutritional deficiencies. When you work on the internal causes of skin concerns, the results are more effective than just applying a cream or ointment and hoping for the best.

Problems with the skin can suggest that the other elimination organs are overloaded, thereby forcing the skin to deal with greater amounts of toxins than it is capable of. Rashes, hives, acne, psoriasis, or eczema are the possible results.

In Chinese medicine, skin problems often indicate lung stress or toxin overload. The approach to diagnosis in traditional Chinese medicine (TCM) is quite different from a Western approach. There are many pathways in the body that carry energy to all the organs, tissues, and cells. The pathway, or meridian, as it is called in Chinese medicine, for the lung also governs the skin. Skin problems are a symptom of a blockage or blockages in the lung meridian. You will learn more about energy and blockages in Chapter 6.

THE LUNGS AND RESPIRATORY SYSTEM

Symptoms such as a chronic cough, runny nose, bronchitis, wheezing, and sinusitis are signs that your body's respiratory system is overloaded with toxins and needs cleansing. The respiratory system enables you to breathe. It includes the nose, sinuses, pharynx, hypopharynx, larynx, vocal cords, trachea, and, of course, the lungs. While all these parts are important, we will focus our attention on the lungs, since they are so vital to life.

Air enters the upper passage of the respiratory system and divides into the two bronchial tubes behind the rib cage, then moves into smaller tubes called bronchioles, until it reaches millions of tiny sacs called alveoli. It is in these sacs that oxygen is extracted and supplied to capillaries in the bloodstream, where it can combine with red blood cells and be carried to every part of your body.

With every exhalation, your lungs work in reverse to release carbon dioxide. The lungs have the greatest exposure to the environment of all our internal organs, making them susceptible to the many air pollutants they come in contact with. Air contains microorganisms, synthetic chemicals, dust, and pollutants, all of which need to be filtered by the lungs.

THE LYMPHATIC SYSTEM

If you are like most people, you have never heard of the lymphatic system. This is quite tragic because it is one of the main systems that encourage efficient detoxification in your body. Efficient detoxification spells vibrant health and healing.

Harvey Diamond, author of *Fit for Life*, describes the lymphatic system as the "number one factor in achieving good health."[9] I agree with him. Yet has any doctor ever told you that your lymphatic system is overloaded when you are experiencing health problems? I doubt it. For that matter, has any doctor, nurse, teacher, or public health official ever even explained to you what the lymphatic system is? Not likely. It is time that someone explained this "number one factor in achieving good health" to you.

The lymphatic system is a complex network of fluid-filled nodes, glands, and tubes that bathe our cells and carry the body's "sewage" away from the tissues to neutralize them. It is comparable to a street-sweeping system throughout your body's tissues. The lymphatic system relies on lymph fluid to suspend toxins, thereby enabling your body to pick up waste that accumulates in every cell in your body, break it down, and get rid of it.

You have three times as much lymph fluid in your body as blood. While blood has the heart to pump it, lymph fluid relies on movement to flow effectively. If you get inadequate exercise or live the life of a couch potato, you can see how this could be a problem. The lymphatic system will not function at its peak. It will be inefficient at eliminating all the toxins that build up in your tissues. These toxins can be waste products of metabolism, fat molecules, and chemical waste that found its way into your body. The result: weight gain, aches and pains, fibromyalgia, or other states of disease. The less you move your body, the more stagnant toxins remain in the lymphatic system, and lymphatic fluid will back up, causing bloating.

Stress plays a role in causing this system to get backed up as well. Ann Louise Gittleman, best-selling author of *The Fat Flush Plan*, states that "the muscles and motion of breathing is a primary way our bodies move lymph, and when we're under stress our breathing becomes shallow." Gittleman suggests that "in many cases, bloated tissue can cause you to swell two extra... sizes. Many experts also believe that a lazy lymphatic system is directly connected to the formation of cellulite because backed up fluid 'sticks' to fat cells."[10]

In addition, bloated tissues prevent cells from properly absorbing oxygen and nutrients. The cells begin to starve and cannot function at their best.

THE BLOODSTREAM AND CARDIOVASCULAR SYSTEM

From the moment we sustain our first scraped knees or cut fingers, we are familiar with blood. What we may not be familiar with, however, is how our bloodstream works to help detoxify our body. Your veins carry fresh oxygenated blood throughout your body to bathe your cells, tissues, and organs in the oxygen that is needed for every function. Your arteries carry toxins to their predetermined exit route in the body. The lymphatic system dumps toxins into your blood after it has swept them up so the blood can carry them to the other detox systems such as the kidneys or liver.

Your heart is the pump that helps push oxygenated blood throughout your body and helps your body deal with the toxins carried by the blood. If you don't get regular exercise to increase your heart rate to boost your blood's circulation, your cells will be deficient in oxygen, and toxins will not be adequately eliminated from your body.

FATTY DEPOSITS

While not officially an organ or a detoxification system, your body stores fatty deposits when it cannot break down and eliminate the toxins to which you are exposed. The same is true of cellulite, particularly if your lymphatic system is not functioning up to par. You may have noticed that many women, even quite fit and athletic ones, suffer from cellulite. You may be one of these women. No matter how hard you try to exercise, the cellulite remains. This is typically because the lymphatic system is not able to eliminate the overwhelming number of toxins to which it is exposed and deposits the extra ones in cellulite or fatty deposits around the body. The more you reduce your exposure to and eliminate excess toxins, the greater your chances of eliminating excess fat and cellulite.

You will learn more about these organs and organ systems in greater detail in Chapters 8 to 11. Throughout *The 4-Week Ultimate Body Detox Plan* you will find herbs, foods, juices, and therapies that target the various organ systems to get them to function far more efficiently.

RATE OF DETOXIFICATION

Everyone is unique, so the same exposure to the same toxins can cause totally different effects. One person may feel as though he is on death's doorstep while another person may feel no symptoms at all. The December 1987 issue of *Discover* magazine reported on ten-month-old fraternal twin girls in Washington, D.C., who had equally high levels of lead in their blood. One girl had many symptoms of lead poisoning such as insomnia, crankiness, and constipation, while the other girl had no symptoms.[11]

Although infants have enzymes in their bodies for detoxification purposes at the time of birth, they are more vulnerable to toxins, partly because they breathe more heavily than adults for their weight, and their detoxification rate is slower than that of adults.[12]

Research shows that people of European descent are less efficient at metabolizing toxins than people of Asian descent. Some people have genetic weaknesses in particular detoxification processes, making them more susceptible to toxins. The efficiency and speed of detoxification are affected by the number and capabilities of the enzymes required for each detoxification process. Enzymes are a particular form of protein found in all living things that speeds up chemical processes. They are required for every function in your body, including digestion, elimination, and detoxification. Without them, life would simply not be possible. Digestion, elimination, and detoxification would not be possible without enzymes. You will learn more about enzymes found in food throughout the rest of this book.

Another factor determining the efficiency of detoxification is nutritional status. This is because your body needs specific vitamins, minerals, and other nutrients to create enzymes or allow them to function. If these nutrients are not found in a person's diet, the enzyme essentially becomes paralyzed or inactive and unable to complete its specific phase of detoxification, leaving a person further susceptible to toxins. For example, as you learned in Chapter 2, people who cannot break down and eliminate pesticides from their bodies are more susceptible to Alzheimer's disease.

The quantity and buildup of toxins in your body is another factor that determines how long it will take to return your detoxification processes to full efficiency. It is similar to what happens to a piece of clothing if you spill grape juice on it but do not wash it for a week: the clothing will be more difficult to clean than if you washed it immediately after staining it.

If you are immensely stressed out on a regular basis, none of your body's functions will be at optimum levels. Also, your body will need to detoxify itself of stress hormones—an added burden as it tries to filter other substances.

Additionally, some synthetic chemicals are foreign to the body, and it may have inefficient or no means to eliminate them effectively. This is not surprising when you consider that there are approximately 500,000 chemicals in use today, according to the Environmental Protection Agency (EPA), and each year more than 5,000 new chemicals are added. There are bound to be some that your body has difficulty eliminating.

The body finds some toxins difficult to eliminate and chooses to absorb them as part of its fatty tissues, allowing them to remain in the body for lengthy periods of time. This obviously slows the process of detoxification down further since the body will also have to eliminate the fat deposits.

An imbalance in the efficiency of various detoxification pathways in your body will result in a slowing of elimination of toxins as well. The process is something like a dammed river. If the water flowing into a dam flows substantially faster than the amount moving through the dam, eventually the water will overflow onto riverbanks and potentially cause flooding. Toxins are comparable to the water flowing through the dam: the process needs to occur in a balanced manner, allowing all organs to complete the tasks they need to before the toxins are sent on to the next organ; otherwise there will be a backlog and potential outpouring of toxins, making you feel lousy and resulting in any number of negative symptoms or disease.

NUTRIENTS REQUIRED FOR DETOXIFICATION

Based on current research, there are many known vitamins, minerals, and other nutrients that are essential for optimum detoxification to take place in your body. Some of the vitamins required include beta carotene (converts to vitamin A), folic acid (vitamin B9), niacin (vitamin B3), pantothenic acid (vitamin B5), riboflavin (vitamin B2), thiamine (vitamin B1), vitamin B12, pyridoxine (vitamin B6), vitamin C, and vitamin E. Your body requires the following minerals for superior detoxification functions: calcium, copper, germanium, iron, magnesium, manganese, molybdenum, selenium, sulphur, and zinc. In addition, other nutrients such as alpha-ketoglutaric acid, chlorophyll, choline, cysteine, d-glucarate, digestive enzymes, fatty acids, glycine, lecithin, l-glutathione, methionine, n-acetyl cysteine, silymarin, and taurine are required for adequate internal cleansing. You need not be familiar with all these nutrients. I include them to help you understand that a diet deficient in nutrients will have detrimental effects on your body's ability to cope with an onslaught of toxins.

Many other nutrients are essential to a properly functioning body, but those listed above are widely recognized to have a specific role in the many functions of detoxification in the digestive tract, liver, kidneys, skin, and other systems. See the following charts to learn about some of the vitamins and minerals that are essential to detoxification and the best food sources in which they are found. You may notice many food sources that are missing from these lists: this is not an oversight. The body varies in its ability to extract and assimilate the nutrients from different foods. For example, calcium is found in milk and other dairy products, but they are not suitable foods for cleansing. In truth, they are not really suitable for human consumption at all. Forget what you read about dairy products providing an excellent source of calcium for your diet. While it is true that they are high in calcium, so is soil in parts of the planet. That does not mean that eating dirt will ensure your body gets adequate calcium, although many young children may have tried this approach.

Yes, it is true that dairy products contain high amounts of calcium. However, the body must digest, utilize, and absorb this calcium to benefit from it. There are many biochemical problems in the way in which dairy products are broken down by the body. What many so-called experts are not considering is some basic biochemistry with respect to the way in which dairy products are *used* by the body or, more accurately, *not used* by the body.

Although dairy foods may be high in calcium when studied in a laboratory, the body does not offer the same conditions as a laboratory. Conversely, the conditions of the body cannot be simulated in a laboratory. In addition, because each person is different, the laboratory cannot account for biochemical individuality.[13]

Dairy products are extremely acid-forming in the body. Acidic blood requires—you guessed it—*calcium* pulled from the bones to neutralize all that acid in the blood. Dr. Robert O. Young, a renowned microbiologist and nutritionist, and co-author Shelley Redford Young state in their recent book, *The pH Miracle: Balance Your Diet, Reclaim Your Health,* "Overacidification of body fluids and tissues underlies *all* disease, and general 'dis-ease' as well." They add, "No matter how many times you were told by teachers and parents to drink your milk, and cute milk moustache ads notwithstanding, the idea that dairy products are healthy is pure hype—a cultural myth. Even if cows lived in some kind of bovine utopia and produced the perfect milk, let's face it: It simply isn't a human food. It is designed for baby cows, whose requirements are far different from those of humans.... No other animal species drinks milk beyond infancy: and certainly not from a species outside their own!"[14]

Harvey Diamond says: "In the same way that we have been conditioned to think of meat whenever the word 'protein' is mentioned, we have also been taught to believe that dairy products are the finest source of calcium, and the best means by which to prevent osteoporosis."[15]

Unfortunately, the high amount of acidity resulting from excessive dairy consumption can pose a problem for detoxification. Besides that, if calcium is being used to neutralize blood acidity, there may be inadequate calcium for the processes of detoxification.

Many nutrients are required for adequate detoxification. The following chart indicates the vitamins and minerals that are most critical. It is by no means a complete list, but it gives you an idea of the importance of obtaining adequate nutrition from your food to ensure healthy detoxification.

Nutrients Required for Detoxification

Vitamins	Some of the Best Food Sources
Beta carotene	Carrots, beets, leafy greens, melon, squash, yams
Folic Acid	Mushrooms, nuts, whole grains, broccoli, asparagus, beans, lettuce, spinach, beet greens, sweet potatoes, leafy greens
Niacin	Avocados, dates, figs, green vegetables, whole grains, brown rice, sunflower seeds
Pantothenic Acid	Green vegetables, beans, kale, cauliflower, peas, sweet potatoes, whole grains, brown rice

Riboflavin	Whole grains, almonds, sunflower seeds, currants, asparagus, broccoli, leafy greens
Vitamin B1 (Thiamine)	Brown rice, nuts, seeds, nut butters, oats, asparagus, beets, leafy greens, plums, raisins
Vitamin B12	Kelp, bananas, peanuts, Concord grapes, sprouts
Vitamin B6 (Pyridoxine)	Bananas, avocados, whole grains, cantaloupe, walnuts, soybeans, peanuts, pecans, leafy greens, green peppers, carrots
Vitamin C	Citrus fruits, apples, strawberries, beet greens, spinach, cabbage, broccoli, cauliflower, kale, tomatoes, sweet potatoes, peppers, papaya, Swiss chard, squash
Vitamin E	Whole grains, Brussels sprouts, leafy greens, spinach, cold-pressed vegetable oils, soybeans, brown rice

Minerals	Some of the Best Food Sources
Calcium	Leafy greens, tofu, soy beans, soy milk, almonds, carob, sesame seeds, tahini, navy beans, walnuts, millet, kelp, carrot juice, oats, and broccoli
Copper	Almonds, peanuts, dried peas and beans, avocados, plums, cherries, citrus fruits, raisins, whole grains, oats, leafy greens
Germanium	Garlic, shiitake mushrooms, onions, whole grains
Iron	Apricots, peaches, bananas, raisins, figs, whole rye, walnuts, kelp, dry beans, leafy greens, asparagus, potatoes

Magnesium	Apples, figs, lemons, peaches, kale, endive, chard, celery, alfalfa sprouts, beet greens, whole grains, brown rice, sesame seeds, sunflower seeds, almonds, honey
Manganese	Nuts, whole grains, spinach, beets, beet greens, Brussels sprouts, peas, kelp, tea, apricots, blueberries, bananas, citrus fruits
Molybdenum	Brown rice, millet, buckwheat, legumes, leafy greens, whole grains
Selenium	Brown rice, soybeans, Brazil nuts, kelp, garlic, mushrooms, pineapple, onions, tomatoes, broccoli
Sulphur	Radish, turnip, onions, celery, horseradish, kale, soybeans, cucumber
Zinc	Sprouted seeds, pumpkin seeds, sunflower seeds, onions, nuts, leafy greens, peas, beets, beet greens

CLEANSING FROM THE INSIDE OUT

The 4-Week Ultimate Body Detox Plan takes a three-fold approach:

1. We will cleanse your body of toxins that have built up in your cells, tissues, organs, and organ systems (this will be discussed in greater detail in Chapter 5).
2. At the same time, we will work to reduce your exposure to further toxins (see below).
3. Once we have achieved results in these two areas, we will help your body to rebuild through proper nutrition and healing therapies.

Toxins affect the body primarily at the cellular level, where symptoms may not be evident. But lack of symptoms is not synonymous with perfect health. By now you have completed "The Detox Quiz" in Chapter 1. So you are aware of the types of symptoms linked with toxins in your body's cells, tissues, organs, and organ systems. The quiz gives you an indication of the most common symptoms and conditions associated with toxins, but toxic buildup in your body can create any symptom. Symptoms are signals from your body that something is wrong and ignoring them can be risky.

Your body strives to restore health in every millisecond you are alive but this can happen only when its specific needs are met. Your body needs enzymes, oxygen, clean water, vitamins and minerals, a proper pH balance, a healthy system of digestion and elimination, electrically charged tissues and cells, healthy emotions, love, and a sense of purpose and fulfilment, among other things. It needs you to stop exposing your body to toxins so that it can eliminate those that have already built up.

WHAT CAN YOU EXPECT WHILE DETOXIFYING?

I have organized *The 4-Week Ultimate Body Detox Plan* to lower your chance of experiencing negative symptoms, but you may still experience some minor ones. Your reaction will depend on how many toxins have accumulated in your body. The more toxins you have, the more likely you will experience some minor symptoms such as fatigue, headaches, or minor body aches; however, they will be short-lived and will soon be replaced with feelings of energy and a reduction of aches and pains you may be living with.

Your body has accumulated many years of toxins that will begin to be pulled out of your tissues, which in the short term means that they will be dumped into your blood to be taken to the most suitable exit route: the liver, the kidneys, the skin, or another detox mechanism in your body. In the short term, the toxins in your blood may create some minor negative symptoms and your organs will have more work to do to eliminate them. That is the reason you will experience some minor discomfort and a decrease in energy while your body uses its energy to eliminate toxins.

Some people should not do a detoxification program. If you are diabetic, pregnant, or nursing or have been diagnosed with a serious medical condition, you should consult your medical or naturopathic doctor or other qualified health practitioner. If you have a history of medical concerns, you should be monitored throughout the detoxification process.

Having said that, most people will experience no negative symptoms at all. This program has been designed to prevent too many toxins from being dumped into your body all at once, instead, releasing them as your detoxification systems can keep up with them. It is also designed to cleanse your intestines and lymphatic systems before targeting the liver, skin, blood, and respiratory systems. In my experience, inadequate bowel function can prevent toxins from being eliminated from your body. Instead, they will be absorbed from your bowels into your blood and be deposited in your tissues, creating a tremendous burden on the lymphatic system and other detoxification systems. By first cleansing the intestinal tract so that toxins are rapidly eliminated from the body, we can prevent new ones from overburdening the lymphatic system.

Afterward, we will focus on each cleansing system, in a sequential order to lessen any negative symptoms and improve the efficiency of each detox mechanism in your body. This will result in improved health as you continue with the program.

HOW TO REDUCE YOUR EXPOSURE TO TOXINS

Before I explain the process we are going to undertake to help your body eliminate the toxins that have built up, it is important to reduce the number of toxins you keep inhaling, ingesting, or absorbing, otherwise the process will be futile. We need to eliminate the toxins that *already* exist in your body without adding too many more. Otherwise, your body's detox systems will be similar to a mouse running in a spinning wheel. They will go nowhere fast.

This part of the plan is as critical as the actual detox process itself. If you continue to increase your body's burden of eliminating toxins by exposing yourself to them in the many ways you learned in Chapter 2, you will have minimal results. It is important to reduce the toxins you eat, drink, inhale, or absorb by tackling the toxins in your foods and beverages; in your home, in the form of cleaning products and furnishings; and in your personal hygiene products and cosmetics.

In the next chapter you will learn additional ways to decrease the toxins you are exposed to in your food and beverages. Before we start with that, begin to lower your toxic exposures by choosing "clean" cleaning and personal-care products. By "clean" I am referring to products that have no synthetic chemicals and unnatural ingredients.

Choosing Cleaning Products

Cleaning products are one of the most common ways to expose your body to toxins, both in the air you breathe on a regular basis and through skin contact. On the positive side of things, changing your household cleaning products is one of the simplest ways to decrease your exposure to harmful toxins immediately. Here are some simple ways to limit your exposure to toxic chemicals in cleaning products:

1. Stop using most commercial brands of cleaning products.
2. Choose natural brands of cleaning products found in most health food stores. (Many of the grocery store "environmentally friendly" cleaning products are not free of toxins that affect people, so avoid them.) Some grocery stores have started including a natural food section within the store. Usually cleaning items found in this section are safer options.

3. Alternatively, you can make your own cleaning products from natural products such as white vinegar, baking soda, and club soda. Baking soda serves as an excellent scouring powder, a polish, and cleaner. It absorbs odours and is a natural fungicide. Aromatherapy oils such as citrus and tea tree have excellent antifungal and antibacterial properties and leave your home smelling fresh and clean. They can be added to natural cleaners. Vinegar removes calcium deposits. Lemon juice removes ink stains on clothes.
4. Avoid so-called air fresheners or potpourri mixes. They are loaded with toxic chemicals.
5. Avoid "natural-like" oils for burning in aromatherapy burners. They are synthetic chemicals and are absolutely not safe. Freshen the air with pure essential oils. Add a drop to your natural cleaning solutions or burn in a potpourri burner.

Choosing Cosmetics and Beauty Products

Stop inundating one of the most important detoxification systems in your body (your skin) by slathering on creams, oils, lotions, cosmetics, deodorants, or other personal-care products that clog your skin. Using products that contain harsh, synthetic ingredients will only prevent your skin from eliminating toxins. It will be working in reverse—absorbing more toxins! Switching to natural hair- and body-care products and cosmetics is a simple and effective way to lessen your body's burden.

Here are some important things to consider when purchasing cosmetics, skin-care, hair-care, and cleansing products:

1. Avoid products that do not list their ingredients on the label. Usually these products are full of nasty ingredients that the manufacturers do not want you to be aware of.
2. Avoid perfumes and colognes and other products that

list "fragrance" on the label. Most contain harmful petro-chemicals and are loaded with hundreds of different toxic ingredients. As I mentioned in Chapter 2, there are over four hundred potential chemicals in this "one" ingredient. If you must wear a scent, choose a natural, high-quality product made with pure essential oils available in health food stores. Be aware of the fragrances contained in cleaning products, shampoos, conditioners, lotions, creams, beauty masks, deo-dorants, cosmetics, and other personal-care products.

3. Avoid products that list FD&C or D&C (Colour) (Number) such as FD&C Red No. 6.

4. Avoid many popular brand deodorants since they contain alumi-num—a heavy metal that has been linked with central nervous system disorders and other illnesses. Make sure the natural one you select says "aluminum-free" or something similar.

5. Beware of most "natural products" that are not sold in health food stores. Many cosmetic manufacturers boldly declare the "natural" status of their products. They may even look and smell natural but may be loaded with toxic chemicals. The word "natural" really does not mean anything, based on the lack of legislation over what "natural" should mean. Unfortunately, salespeople and advertisements throw the word "natural" around quite prolifically. In some cases, the claim is true, but in most it is not.

6. Start purchasing your hair products, deodorants, moistur-izers, facial masks, hand and body lotions, soaps, bath and shower gels, hairsprays, hair gels, and cosmetics at a health food store.

7. Use natural hair dyes or hennas found in health food stores. Many hair salons claim their products are "natural" but a quick look at the ingredient list reveals items I would never want to come in contact with.

Become conscious of the cleaning, beauty, and hygiene products you use on a regular basis. This will prevent the addition of new toxins to your body. In the coming chapters, you will learn how to eliminate the toxic buildup that your body is facing.

In this chapter you learned

- Detoxification helps create greater energy, balance weight, eliminate negative symptoms, reduce cellulite, and much more
- The major detoxification organs and systems, such as the kidneys and urinary tract, intestines, liver, gallbladder, lymphatic system, and lungs, help your body eliminate toxins and toxic buildup
- You can immediately start eliminating toxins from your environment by choosing healthier cleaning and personal-care products

References

1. Kim Erickson, "On the Fast Track," *Herbs for Health*, March/April 2004, p. 33.

2. Erickson, "On the Fast Track," p. 33.

3. Erickson, "On the Fast Track," p. 33.

4. Erickson, "On the Fast Track," p. 33.

5. Erickson, "On the Fast Track," p. 33.

6. Erickson, "On the Fast Track," p. 33.

7. Xandria Williams, *The Herbal Detox Plan* (Carlsbad, CA: Hay House, 2004), p. 82.

8. Williams, *The Herbal Detox Plan*, p. 82.

9. Michelle Schoffro Cook, "The Secret of Great Health—An Interview with Best-Selling Author Harvey Diamond," April 2003.

10. Jillian Boyle, "Is Lymphatic Stress the Reason You're Fat? Bloated? Hungry for Junk Food?" *Woman's World*, March 2, 2004.

11. Jacqueline Krohn and Frances Taylor, *Natural Detoxification: A Practical Encyclopedia* (Vancouver, BC: Hartley & Marks Publishers, 2000), p. 30.

12. *Natural Detoxification: A Practical Encyclopedia.*

13. Michelle Schoffro Cook, *Healing Injuries the Natural Way* (Toronto, ON: Your Health Press, 2004).

14. Robert O. Young and Shelley Redford Young, *The pH Miracle: Balance Your Diet, Reclaim Your Health*, p. 77.

15. Harvey Diamond, *The Fit for Life Solution* (St. Paul, MN: Dragon Door Publications, Inc., 2002).

CHAPTER 5

The 4-Week Ultimate Body Detox Plan

What separates two people most profoundly is a different sense and degree of cleanliness.
Friedrich Nietzsche

In this chapter you will learn
- How to decrease your exposure to toxins in your foods and beverages
- How to effectively eliminate toxic buildup in your intestines, liver, kidneys, lungs, blood, lymph, skin, and fatty deposits
- The best order in which to cleanse your body's detoxification organs

Cleansing your body of toxic buildup at the cellular, tissue, and organ levels as well as emotional and energetic levels, can mean the difference between fatigue and energy, pain and being pain-free, and having poor health or having great health.

Now that you are aware of the many toxins you are regularly exposed to, ways to lower your exposure in your home and personal-care products, and why it is essential to detoxify your body, it is time to get down to eliminating toxins from the foods you eat and start to cleanse your body of the toxins that may have built up over the years.

Although you can never totally eliminate toxins from your food, beverages, air, metabolic processes, and other exposures, it does not mean that you should sit back and wait for disease to strike. It means that not only is it important to minimize your exposure to toxins by choosing healthier options, it is essential to get and keep your detoxified organs and systems functioning optimally. In that way, they are better prepared to remove the toxins to which they are exposed and eliminate them before they can damage your body.

The 4-Week Ultimate Body Detox Plan uses many forms of natural therapies to restore your body's functioning: nutritional therapy (the use of food as medicine), herbal therapy, nutritional supplementation, juicing, hydrotherapy (the use of water to heal the body), exercise, homeopathy, Bach flower therapy, aromatherapy, breath work, sound therapy, meditation, energy medicine, body work, massage and more.

The 4-Week Ultimate Body Detox Plan is designed to provide thorough cleansing, much deeper than many of the cleansing programs currently available in book form and much more thorough than most of the ready-made supplement programs available in stores. Using the above therapies, we will cleanse your intestinal tract, kidneys, lymphatic system, liver, gallbladder, blood, lungs, skin, and fatty deposits (yes, even cellulite).

For most people, the program consists of four weeks; however, if you are quite overweight, have been exposed to large amounts of toxins, or are experiencing severe ill effects of toxins (such as fibromyalgia, chronic fatigue syndrome, lupus, multiple sclerosis, cancer, or another serious disorder), you will likely need to spend more time detoxifying. The amount of time varies from person to person and largely depends on the nature of the toxic exposure, the amount you are overweight, the volume of toxins in your body, and the length of time you have been ill. Do not be discouraged, however, since if you fall into this category, you will likely reap the greatest rewards from following *The 4-Week Ultimate Body Detox Plan.*

Although each phase is designed to be one week long, you will be guided from one step to the next so you know when it is time to move to the next phase. The program takes some effort but is still easy enough to fit into most people's lives.

Each week builds on the last week. For example, in week one you will begin to cleanse your kidneys and urinary and intestinal tracts. During week two, you will begin to focus more attention on the lymphatic system, but will still be cleansing the kidneys and urinary and intestinal tracts. This week will also begin to help with cellulite cleansing. During week three, we will add attention to the liver and gallbladder. This will also help with your body's ability to break down any fat stores that may be leading to being overweight. And, finally, in week four we will shift our attention to the blood and circulatory system, lungs and respiratory tract, and skin.

There are some things that are required throughout the program for the best results. By now, it is assumed that you have already started switching your household cleaning products as well as your personal-care products. There are many additional ways to decrease your intake of toxins so you obtain maximum benefits from *The 4-Week Ultimate Body Detox Plan.*

ESSENTIALS OF *THE 4-WEEK ULTIMATE BODY DETOX PLAN*

The following parts of *The 4-Week Ultimate Body Detox Plan* are common to Phases 1, 2, 3, and 4. Over the next four weeks, you will need to do the following:

Drink plenty of purified water (at least eight to ten cups (250 mL cups) per day). Add Cellfood® (see resources) to three cups per day. This is essential throughout the program because it helps to flush out the many toxins that will be stirred up and eliminated from fat stores and organs in your body. Cellfood® speeds detoxification, particularly of the blood, lymphatic system, and kidneys. It aids water absorption at the cellular level and, unlike many other oxygen supplements, provides valuable nutrients, oxygen, and enzymes needed for healthy detoxification.

It is important that you eat plenty of raw fruits and vegetables on this program. The enzymes, fibre, water content, vitamins, minerals, and high-quality protein that fruits and vegetables provide will help ensure that your nutritional needs are met, particularly since the detox mechanisms in your body have specific requirements. I highly recommend that you eat organic produce wherever possible since you are trying to eliminate toxins from your body. Eating conventionally grown produce increases your exposure to pesticides and other toxins, the very ones that we are trying to decrease your exposure to and eliminate from your body.

Thoroughly wash fruits and vegetables before consuming them to eliminate any microorganisms that may be present. Also, if you are unable to buy organic produce, scrubbing your conventionally grown fruits and vegetables thoroughly will help to reduce your exposure to pesticides and pathogens such as bacteria, fungi, mould, etc.

Meat is very acidic and requires tremendous energy to digest. I recommend avoiding meat altogether for this cleanse; however, if you simply must have some, limit your consumption to one serving per week maximum. If you do choose to eat meat, it is imperative that you purchase only organic meat or poultry. Animals are fed hormones, antibiotics, and other medications to fatten them and to supposedly keep them healthy. These toxins become concentrated in the meat we eat. So if you must eat some meat or poultry throughout your cleanse, eat organic meat a maximum of one time per week. This will not only be better for your body, but better for the planet as well.

Limit your consumption of sweets. You can use as sweeteners small amounts of stevia (a herb that is naturally one thousand times sweeter than sugar without the harmful effects on your blood sugar levels and your pancreas); raw, unfiltered honey; pure maple syrup; or raw sugar. Raw sugar is not the same as turbinado, demerara, or brown sugar. The latter three are refined white sugar to which molasses is added. Avoid them. Other sugars to avoid include molasses, beet sugar, date sugar, corn syrup, glucose, fructose (this is fruit sugar that has been heavily refined), sucrose, maltose, or anything on a food label that reads "-ose." They are just as damaging to your body as white sugar. Of course, your best option is fruit. Forget what Dr. Atkins tells you about fruit. Fruit is the most cleansing of all foods. Throughout this program, you will be eating plenty of fruit. If you believe you cannot tolerate fruit because it gives you indigestion, you may be eating it at the wrong time. Fruit is rapidly digested and doesn't need to be digested in the stomach like other foods. If you eat fruit after eating foods that need to be digested in the stomach (all other foods), all the food, including the fruit, will sit together and begin to ferment. This will cause all sorts of digestive troubles. However, if you eat fruit on an empty stomach, you will likely be able to tolerate it without any discomfort. You will learn more about fruit consumption and its effects on cleansing in a moment. Be aware that soft drinks, sweetened juices, fruit punch, and other beverages contain concentrated sweeteners that are not permitted on this program.

Those that are sweetened with fruit juice or fruit purée are still too concentrated and cause rapid blood sugar fluctuations.

Avoid *all* synthetic sweeteners, including Nutrasweet, saccharin, aspartame, and any of the sweeteners that slick marketers claim "go through your body undigested" or "contain zero calories." The diseases that have been linked with these sweeteners are pages long. Really. If you are to experience the benefits of this program, avoiding chemical sweeteners is essential.

Avoid alcohol, tobacco, and recreational drugs throughout this program. If you absolutely cannot stop smoking, you will still get some benefits from following the program; however, they will be much greater if you choose to quit smoking. If you are just not ready to kick the habit, detoxifying your body can help reduce cravings so following the program may help you to quit eventually.

Use prescription and over-the-counter drugs only when essential. Consult a medical doctor before discontinuing any medications, however, since discontinuing some medications can have detrimental effects and potentially be fatal. If your doctor says you can stop medications, he or she may need to monitor you. But think twice before popping a pill for pain or indigestion or some other common malady and take them only if they are absolutely essential.

Exercise regularly away from high-traffic or high-pollution areas. Walking or running near highways or busy roads, for example, exposes your body to large amounts of petrochemicals and other pollutants at a time when your breathing is deeper than normal. I recommend rebounding—bouncing on a mini trampoline. You'll learn more about this in Chapter 6. Rebounding not only offers a good cardiovascular workout, it helps the lymphatic system to flow, resulting in fewer toxins. Rebounding reduces any strain on joints that you may experience with other forms of activities. In addition, I also recommend a brisk thirty-minute walk every day, five days a week, preferably outdoors so you can get some fresh air.

Avoid using pesticides and herbicides indoors or outdoors, and limit your exposure to areas that have been sprayed. Many parks, golf courses, and even neighbours' lawns are sprayed with pesticides. Keep your exposure in these areas to a minimum while detoxifying. It is a good idea to continue this practice as best you are able even after you are finished *The 4-Week Ultimate Body Detox Plan*.

By now, you should have switched to natural cleaning products devoid of potentially toxic synthetic chemicals for your home. Continue this practice throughout the program and, preferably, permanently.

Eat only fresh foods. Avoid all processed, packaged, or fast foods. Prepared, packaged, and fast foods are typically loaded with chemical preservatives, colours, and other additives that are dangerous at any time, but must be avoided for *The 4-Week Ultimate Body Detox Plan* if you are to see results from your efforts.

Do not eat fried foods. That includes french fries, onion rings, potato chips, nachos, etc.

Avoid margarine and hydrogenated fats like the plague. As you learned in Chapter 2, margarine is highly toxic. I cannot, in good faith, call it food. It has been chemically altered so severely that it is no longer food. It is linked with so many diseases, including cancer, that it really should be banned from human consumption. Hydrogenated fats include margarine, shortening, lard, or products made with them such as cookies, pies, packaged foods, and buns.

Avoid all dairy products and foods made with them. They are mucus-forming and tend to clog the body's detoxification systems. In addition, they tend to be quite acidic once they begin to be digested. Most people are sensitive to dairy products but are not aware of this sensitivity. It may show up as digestive difficulties, bloating, cramping, seasonal allergies, joint or muscle pain, arthritis, and many other symptoms and disorders. Dairy products include butter, milk, yogurt, sour cream, cheese, and cottage cheese. Be aware that dairy products disguise themselves in many other foods such as baked goods, pasta sauces, desserts, and soups.

Do not use salt. Moderate use of Celtic sea salt is allowed but go easy with it. Also, be aware that Celtic sea salt is not the same as sea salt. Celtic sea salt looks slightly damp and has a greyish colour. In addition to the mineral sodium, it contains many other minerals and trace minerals that are necessary for great health.

Refrain from eating wheat products. Wheat, even whole wheat, is very acidifying and can counter the benefits of the program. Wheat products include pastas, couscous, pastries, and breads. Instead, opt for spelt, kamut, brown rice, or other whole-grain breads that do not contain any white flour. You can also eat brown rice, millet, oatmeal, wild rice, and other whole grains on this program. Recipes for these foods are presented later in this book.

To help you remember these principles, I have provided a summary of foods and other items to avoid:

- Meat, poultry, and fish—you can eat them again after the detox is done
- All refined sweeteners and sweetened foods. Look for "-ose" and other forms of sweeteners on ingredient lists
- All synthetic sweeteners (Nutrasweet, saccharin, aspartame, etc.)
- Alcohol, tobacco, and recreational drugs
- Prescription and over-the-counter drugs except when they have been prescribed by a physician
- Indoor and outdoor pesticides and chemical fertilizers
- Cleaning products full of synthetic chemicals
- Margarine and all baked goods made with it
- Dairy products and foods made with butter, cheese, yogurt, cottage cheese, sour cream, milk, and other dairy products
- Fried foods: french fries, onion rings, potato chips, nachos, etc.
- Salt (use Celtic sea salt instead and limit sodium intake. Note: Celtic sea salt is not the same as sea salt)

- All food additives (colours, flavour enhancers, stabilizers, preservatives, etc.)
- All wheat products (wheat, even whole wheat, is very acidifying and can counter the benefits of the program)
- Coffee and black tea (green tea and herbal teas are permitted)
- All soft drinks, sweetened juices, fruit punch, and other sweetened or carbonated beverages

Here is a summary of some of the important foods to eat and healthy practices to incorporate into your life:
- Drink plenty of purified water (eight to ten cups per day minimum)
- Eat plenty of fresh fruits and vegetables (organic as much as possible)
- Wash fruits and vegetables thoroughly before consuming
- Exercise regularly away from high-traffic or high-pollution areas
- Eat only fresh foods; avoid all prepared, packaged, or fast foods

The above principles are critical to the success of the whole program. It is important that you stick with them for the next four weeks. To people whose lives revolve around unhealthy habits, that may seem difficult. Remember this is only four weeks of your life, and those weeks could have the most profound effect on your health. Besides, developing healthy habits may take time. It took many years to develop whatever unhealthy habits you have.

OPTIMUM CLEANSING FOODS
Some foods are better detoxifiers than others. Fruits and some vegetables are perfect cleansers for the body. That does not mean that you should eat only these foods for the next four weeks. There are many other great cleansing foods. The key to attaining the best

results is variety. Choose some of the top twenty-five cleansing foods below to include in your daily diet, but choose others as well. Here are my picks for some of the best internal cleansing foods:

Michelle's Top 25 Cleansing Foods

Almonds—are high in fibre, calcium, and usable protein and help stabilize blood sugar.

Apples—are high in pectin, which helps cleanse the intestines and binds to heavy metals. They lower cholesterol and contain anti-cancer, antibacterial, antiviral, and anti-inflammatory properties. Pectin also helps the body excrete food additives, including tartrazine, a synthetic chemical used in the food industry that has been linked to hyperactivity, migraines, and asthma in children.[1]

Artichokes—increase bile production. Bile helps the intestines eliminate toxins from the body. They also contain a substance that helps the liver break down fatty acids, lightening its immense load.

Avocados—lower cholesterol and dilate blood vessels while blocking artery-destroying toxicity. Avocados contain a nutrient called glutathione, which blocks at least thirty different carcinogens while helping the liver detoxify synthetic chemicals. Researchers at the University of Michigan found that elderly people who had high levels of glutathione were healthier and less likely to suffer from arthritis.[2]

Bananas—soothe and strengthen the stomach while offering plenty of minerals needed for optimal cleansing. The mineral potassium, which is found in plentiful amounts in bananas, helps regulate fluid in the body and reduce fluid buildup in tissues. Excess fluid in the tissues means more stored toxins. Bananas also have antibiotic activity to help kill harmful bacteria residing in the intestines.

Beets—contain a unique mixture of natural plant chemicals (phytochemicals) and minerals that make them superb fighters of infection, blood purifiers, and liver cleansers. They also help boost the body's cellular intake of oxygen, making beets excellent overall body cleansers. Aphrodite, according to legend, ate beets to retain her beauty. She was definitely on to a good thing since beets, in addition to all the benefits listed above, also help stabilize the blood's acid-alkaline balance (pH).

Blueberries—contain natural aspirin that helps reduce the tissue-damaging effects of chronic inflammation, while reducing pain. Blueberries also act as an antibiotic by blocking bacteria in the urinary tract, thereby helping to prevent infections. They also have antiviral properties.

Cabbage—contains numerous anti-cancer and antioxidant compounds and helps the liver break down excess hormones. Cabbage also cleanses the digestive tract and soothes the stomach, which could in part be due to its antibacterial and antiviral properties. Cruciferous vegetables such as cabbage, kale, and spinach demonstrate powerful detoxification activity, including neutralizing some of the damaging compounds found in cigarette smoke (and second-hand smoke). They also contain a compound that helps the liver produce adequate amounts of enzymes for detoxification.

Carrots—contain large amounts of alpha- and beta-carotene, vitamin A precursors, as well as antioxidants, which help protect the body from cellular damage. Carrots seem to cleanse the body of heavy metals, reduce cholesterol levels in the blood, and promote cardiovascular health.

Celery and Celery Seeds—an excellent blood cleanser that helps lower high blood pressure, celery also contains many different anti-cancer compounds that help eliminate cancerous cells from the body. Celery seeds contain over twenty anti-inflammatory substances. They are particularly good for detoxifying substances found in cigarette smoke.

Cherries—contain natural aspirin that helps detoxify inflammation-related substances in the body's tissues and joints. Cherries also contain pectin, which helps to clean up heavy metals, synthetic chemicals disguised as food additives, cholesterol, and buildup in the intestines.

Cranberries—have powerful antibiotic and antiviral substances to help the body cleanse harmful bacteria and viruses from the urinary tract.

Flaxseeds and Flaxseed Oil—are loaded with essential fatty acids, particularly the omega-3s. They are essential for many cleansing functions and maintaining a healthy immune system. They are also critical to maintaining a healthy brain. The health of every cell in your body is dependent on getting adequate amounts of essential fatty acids.

Garlic—helps cleanse harmful bacteria, intestinal parasites, and viruses from the body, especially from the blood and intestines. It also helps cleanse buildup from the arteries and lowers blood pressure. Garlic has anti-cancer and antioxidant properties that help detoxify the body of harmful substances. It also helps cleanse the respiratory tract by expelling mucous buildup in the lungs and sinuses. I am referring to fresh garlic, not garlic powder, which has virtually none of the above properties. Try to eat at least a clove or two per day. Raw is best but cooked garlic is often easier for those of us with sensitive stomachs.

Grapefruit—contains pectin fibre that binds to cholesterol, thereby helping to remove arterial buildup and cleanse the blood. Pectin also binds to heavy metals and helps escort them out of the body. Grapefruit also has anti-cancer properties and helps particularly to protect against stomach and pancreatic cancer. Grapefruit contains powerful antioxidants that help protect the body's cells from damage. It also has antiviral compounds that cleanse harmful viruses out of the body. Grapefruit is an excellent intestinal and liver detoxifier.

Kale—contains powerful anti-cancer and antioxidant compounds that help cleanse the body of harmful substances. It is also high in fibre, which helps cleanse the intestinal tract. Like cabbage, kale helps neutralize compounds found in cigarette smoke and contains a substance that jump-starts the liver's production of cleansing enzymes.

Legumes—are loaded with fibre that helps lower cholesterol, cleanse the intestines, and regulate blood sugar levels. Legumes also help protect the body against cancer.

Lemons—are the best liver detoxifiers. In addition, they contain high amounts of vitamin C, a vitamin needed by the body to make a substance called glutathione. Glutathione helps ensure that phase 2 liver detoxification keeps pace with phase 1, thereby reducing the likelihood of negative effects from environmental chemicals. Vitamin C and other antioxidants found in lemons are integral to warding off cancer, and fighting the effects of pollution and cell damage. They also help our adrenal glands—two triangular-shaped glands that sit atop the kidneys—manage the effects of stress.

Olive Oil—helps cleanse and protect the arteries from plaque build-up while lowering LDL cholesterol (often referred to as the harmful cholesterol) without lowering HDL cholesterol. Olive oil also helps lower blood pressure and regulates blood sugar. In addition, it is a powerful antioxidant and, in some studies, shows anti-cancer activity.

Onions—demonstrate powerful antioxidant and anti-cancer activity. Onions also thin and cleanse the blood and lower LDL cholesterol without lowering HDL cholesterol. Onions also help detoxify the respiratory tract and fight asthma, bronchitis, hay fever, and diabetes. Onions help cleanse the body of viruses and the intestines of harmful bacteria.

Raspberries—have antiviral and anti-cancer properties. These delicious berries also contain natural aspirin that helps fight pain and inflammation in the body, and cleanse the tissues of toxins.

Seaweed—could be the most underrated vegetable in the Western world. Studies at McGill University in Montreal showed that seaweeds bind to radioactive waste in the body.[3] Radioactive waste can find its way into the body through some medical tests or through food that has been grown where water or soil is contaminated. Seaweed also binds to heavy metals to help eliminate them from the body. In addition, it is a powerhouse of minerals and trace minerals.

Spinach—similar to cabbage and kale, spinach helps the body neutralize harmful substances found in cigarette smoke. Spinach also contains glucosinolates, which stimulates the liver's production of cleansing enzymes.

Watercress—increases detoxification enzymes in the body and acts on cancer cells in the body. In a study at the Norwich Food Research Centre in the United Kingdom, smokers who were given 170 grams of watercress per day eliminated higher than average amounts of carcinogens in their urine, thereby eliminating them from their body.

Watermelon—is a good source of an important liver-cleansing substance called glutathione. It helps to ensure that both phases of detoxification within the liver continue at the same speed, thereby preventing toxic buildup in the liver.

There are many other excellent cleansing foods. This list is by no means comprehensive. Eating a variety of fresh fruits and vegetables offers the best results for detoxifying your body.

SUPPLEMENTING YOUR CLEANSING EFFORTS

Many cleansing programs will ask you to pop twenty, thirty, forty, or more pills per day. All these pills need to be broken down by your digestive tract and liver and absorbed into the bloodstream through the walls of the intestines. I find that taking too many nutritional supplements during a cleanse defeats the point: they make organs· such as the liver work extra hard instead of supporting them in their functions. In addition, if your intestines are clogged, you will reap minimal, if any, benefit from them anyway. Not to mention that buying twelve types of supplements or more can become expensive.

Here are the supplements everyone should be taking throughout the cleanse and may wish to continue after the cleanse is over.

They include:

- A high-quality multivitamin and mineral every day
- A high-quality full-spectrum digestive enzyme with every meal
- A potent flora supplement every morning
- A high-quality green food supplement daily
- Cellfood®, a natural oxygen and nutritional supplement

When I say "high-quality" supplements, please know that I am not referring to the cheap brands that may be popular but are primarily made up of synthetic chemicals. I am suggesting supplements that are derived from foods. Many pharmacy and health food store brands are synthetic and offer very little nutritional or health value.

A high-quality multivitamin and mineral will help ensure that your body has the nutrients it needs to detoxify. As you recall from the last chapter, many vitamins and minerals are essential to the many cleansing functions in your body. If you are deficient in them, your cleansing efforts will suffer. This supplement is best taken with food, at breakfast or lunch.

Take a high-quality full-spectrum digestive enzyme with every meal. It will help your body digest the foods you are eating. Ideally, our food comes with its own enzymes to help with digestion, but these enzymes are destroyed with cooking and processing, although you will be avoiding processed foods for the next four weeks. A full-spectrum enzyme includes enzymes that help digest starches, natural sugars, fibre, protein, and fats found in foods. Usually it will include protease (ideally, several types), amylase, lipase, cellulase, peptidase, maltase, lactase, and invertase. Most people have depleted their own supplies of digestive enzymes by eating a highly cooked and heavily processed diet. This supplement will help your body break down the foods you eat. Take one or two capsules or tablets with every meal (breakfast, lunch, and dinner).

Every morning, take a flora supplement. This is to replenish the healthy bacteria that are needed in your intestines to keep less healthy strains in check, to assist with normal bowel movements, and to help nutrients move through the intestinal walls. There are many names for this type of supplement, but ideally they will contain *Lactobacillus acidophilus* and *Bifidobacterium*. These are both healthy strains of natural flora found in healthy intestines. One works best in the small intestine while the other functions ideally in the large intestine. A formula that contains both is preferred. You can take this ten minutes after taking your warm lemon water in the morning. Take one-half to one teaspoon in pure, unchlorinated water. Chlorine kills the bacteria. Alternatively, take the number of capsules or tablets recommended on the product label.

A green food supplement helps supply our bodies with additional nutrients, chlorophyll (the green colour in plants), and phytochemicals found in green foods. It will greatly assist with cleansing. The chlorophyll in green foods and green food supplements helps our bodies make fresh, new, and healthy cells, especially blood cells. Many different green food supplements are available, taken from barley, alfalfa, chlorella, spirulina, and other green foods, or a combination of these. Make sure that the one you select is free of preservatives and artificial sweeteners (the natural plant sweetener, stevia, is fine) and is processed at low temperatures to maintain the integrity of the enzymes naturally present in these foods. The amount you will take will depend on the type of green food supplement you choose. You can have a mid-morning or mid-afternoon fruit smoothie and include a scoop of your green food supplement in it. Follow the amounts suggested on the package. Cellfood® is an unique cell-oxygenating liquid formula that delivers oxygen, 78 trace minerals, 34 enzymes, 17 amino acids and electrolytes to the body's cells.

During *The 4-Week Ultimate Body Detox*, we will work together to help restore balance to your body on many levels, including biochemically, electrically (yes, your body is electric—your nerves carry electrical signals throughout your body and every cell in your body conducts electricity), emotionally, energetically, enzymatically, hormonally, magnetically (yes, your body also has magnetic properties), biologically, nutritionally, psychologically, and spiritually.

We will be working holistically, which simply means we'll be working on the various aspects that make you whole: your body, mind, emotions, and spirit. Many programs claim to be holistic but work only on your physical aspects.

Throughout the program you will follow certain daily patterns, although other activities and foods will be added as we go along. These initial eating and lifestyle patterns should be continued throughout the program. Once you get used to them, they are quite simple and you may even wish to continue them as part of your long-term health plan. They are excellent habits to make and will be a great start toward good health for a lifetime.

Keep in mind that we have many ingrained habits and patterns that we have learned over our lifetimes. Changing these habits so you can form new ones may take time, patience, and some initial effort, at least until they become ingrained. Few people were experts at riding their bicycles from the first moment they leapt onto them. More likely, learning to ride a bike took practice, determination, and diligence. Commit to making positive change in your life by breaking old habits and making new ones. You will be immensely happy you did.

I will recommend various herbs and natural remedies throughout the program; however, unlike many detox programs, this one will not have you swallowing fistfuls of pills. I have selected several of the most important herbal and nutritional remedies for the program. If you need additional help with a particular phase of detoxification, I have provided a more thorough list of remedies in Chapters 8 to 11. The natural remedies found in these chapters are by no means essential to the program. They are provided as an adjunct should you require further cleansing.

Organizing Your Day on
The 4-Week Ultimate Body Detox Plan

Start with the fresh juice of half a lemon squeezed into warm, pure water first thing upon rising in the morning. This helps to stimulate your bowels to eliminate the waste products that may have built up in your intestinal tract. It also helps to balance your blood pH. In other words, it reduces the acidity of your blood. This is essential because pain and disease thrive in acidic blood. The simple act of neutralizing the acidity helps lessen pain and decrease any harmful pathogens that reside in your body. Also, the act of detoxifying stirs up toxins that are predominantly acidic.

You may be thinking, "But lemons are so acidic, how can they possibly alkalize my blood?" Lemons *are* acidic, but when they are metabolized in your body, they have an immensely alkalizing effect.

So it is critical to alkalize your body to counter the effects of the toxins. If toxins remain in your intestines for too long, they will be reabsorbed into your bloodstream, where they need to be filtered by your already overburdened liver and kidneys, and may eventually be deposited in your tissues and fatty deposits, particularly as cellulite in women.

From a holistic medicine viewpoint, cellulite is the result of irregular bowel movements, from holding back urges to eliminate stools, and from a sluggish lymphatic system. Correct these irregularities, and cellulite will typically melt away. That is one of our goals on this program. You will learn more about getting rid of cellulite as we proceed further.

After drinking your lemon water, it is time to skin brush (see Chapter 6 to learn how). It is a simple technique that requires a natural-bristle brush that can be found at many health food stores and spas. It takes less than one minute to do and really stimulates your lymphatic system and improves blood circulation.

If you make time in the morning to exercise, this is the ideal time to rebound. This exercise is one of the most effective ways to get your lymphatic system moving without straining your joints. The mini trampoline absorbs much of the shock to your joints. The bouncing action forces the millions of one-way valves in the lymphatic system to open expansively. According to Morton Walker, podiatrist and author of the book *Jumping for Health*, this action increases the lymph flow up to fourteen times greater than it would otherwise flow. See Chapter 6 to learn the most effective rebounding exercise to incorporate into your detox plan.

After drinking lemon water and rebounding, drink one teaspoon each of psyllium husks and pectin in one and a half cups of pure water or unsweetened juice with no preservatives or additives. The type of juice may vary from week to week. For example, during Phases 1 and 2, you will be adding this fibre to pure, unsweetened cranberry juice (see below).

Psyllium is the seed of a grain grown in India. It makes an excellent intestinal cleanser since it softens (if needed) and adds bulk to the stool. Because it thickens quickly, it is essential to drink it immediately after mixing psyllium with water or juice. Metamucil is one example of a psyllium product but I recommend one that is less heavily processed.

Pectin is a special type of fibre usually extracted from apples. You take it by stirring a teaspoonful or two into a glass of juice or take it in capsule form. Be sure to drink at least one cup of juice or water to ensure you are getting adequate liquid. Pectin binds to heavy metals in the bloodstream and helps flush them out via the liver, according to Nan Kathryn Fuchs, a nutrition researcher.[4]

Based on research from California's Amitabha Medical Center, five grams of pectin daily is enough to flush almost 70 percent of heavy metals out of most people's bodies within months.

According to additional research, a pectin-rich diet may decrease total cholesterol by 12 percent and lower the potentially harmful LDL cholesterol by 15 percent. According to experts, lowering cholesterol by this amount can cut your risk of heart disease by 25 percent.

A recent study found that pectin also attaches itself to cancer cells, thereby preventing up to 95 percent of them from developing into full-blown tumours. Studies in California indicate that taking fourteen grams of pectin daily may help prevent lung, skin, and prostate cancers from spreading.

I highly recommend that most people continue supplementing their diet for at least several months after they have finished *The 4-Week Ultimate Body Detox* for maximum benefits. After that, continue to eat foods high in pectin to help maintain your results. These foods include apples, bananas, beets, cabbage, carrots, citrus fruits, dried peas, and okra.

Eat fruit and fresh fruit juice all morning. If you are drinking fruit juice, do not drink bottled or canned juice. All the enzymes have been destroyed in these types of juices; in addition, they have been heated to high temperatures, a process called pasteurization, to preserve them. This process turns alkaline juice into an acidic one. During the detoxification process, we are trying to reduce the quantity of acidic foods in your diet, to better enable your body to cleanse and heal. You can drink freshly squeezed grapefruit or orange juice. These are simple to make with an electric citrus juicer or by peeling the fruits and blending them in a blender. You can also drink fresh fruit juices made in an electric juicer. Whatever type of juice you choose, dilute it 1:1 with purified water.

You can also eat fresh fruit all morning. Try to mix up the variety you choose to extract a broad range of enzymes, vitamins, minerals, and phytochemicals (powerful natural plant chemicals). This does not mean that you forgo food for several hours, because it can cause blood sugar fluctuations that we are trying to avoid. Instead, every half hour or hour, eat more fruit throughout the morning. You can also make delicious smoothies with just fresh fruit and frozen bananas and a little water. You'll find some of my favourite smoothie and juice recipes later in this book to get you started, but feel free to try other combinations. The important factors to remember are these: fresh or frozen, raw, and variety.

Use this opportunity to try different fruits that you may not have been exposed to in the past. Some nutritional powerhouses include papayas, mangoes, blueberries, raspberries, blackberries, strawberries, pineapple, kiwi, grapes, apples, pears, cherries, and avocado. This is certainly not an exhaustive list. Feel free to try others. Do not worry about calories or quantity. Eat as much as you like until you feel full, then stop. When you feel hungry again or within two hours, eat more fruit until at least noon. You can continue if you would like or you can have lunch.

Wait at least twenty minutes after you have eaten your last piece of fruit before having lunch. If you wish to eat fruit again later in the day, wait until two to three hours have passed since you ate grains, legumes, meat (if you choose to eat it), or another type of food.

Fruits are optimum detoxifiers when eaten on an empty stomach. Fruit starts to be digested in the mouth so it is critical that you chew it well. This allows it to mingle with digestive juices secreted in the mouth. Then it travels through the digestive tract. Typically within half an hour, fruit leaves the stomach and enters the intestines, where it offers its natural sugars, enzymes, vitamins, and minerals for cleansing and healing. Many people complain that fruit gives them gas or indigestion. The primary reason for this is inadequate chewing to break down the food sufficiently. Another reason is that people often eat fruit after other foods that take significantly longer to digest in the stomach. Eating fruit with or after other types of foods causes everything to sit in the stomach and begin to putrefy. This putrefaction causes gas, bloating, and indigestion. During *The 4-Week Ultimate Body Detox Plan* (and afterward, I hope) you will eat fruit on an empty stomach to benefit from its cleansing properties and avoid digestive discomforts.

Drink three cups of pure water with eight drops of Cellfood® per cup on an empty stomach throughout the day. Drink an additional five to seven cups of pure water on an empty stomach throughout the day.

For lunch, eat a large green salad. Green means that it actually resembles the colour green. That excludes iceberg lettuce, which really looks more like white. You can eat mesclun (also known as spring mix), romaine (sometimes called cos), arugula, dandelion greens, Boston lettuce, mustard greens, beet greens, watercress, spinach, frisée, red leaf lettuce or radicchio (which are the exceptions to the "green rule" since they are red). If you choose dandelion greens, organic are best. Do not harvest them from a lawn that has been sprayed with pesticides or synthetic fertilizers and certainly do not pick them if they are growing near roads. Add as many other vegetables as you would like to create variety.

Choose from a wide range of salad dressings listed in this book or from cold-pressed vegetable, nut, or seed oils and a squeeze of fresh lemon juice or apple cider vinegar. (Make sure it has not been pasteurised. It should have some sediment in the bottom or state on the label that it contains the "mother" or "live culture.") Do not use bottled dressings from the grocery store. They are typically packed with preservatives, emulsifiers, sugar, and other junk that will work against your best cleansing efforts. You will find many delicious recipes for dressings in this book that take only minutes to prepare and can be stored in the refrigerator for use throughout the week.

You will also have a large meal-sized salad with dinner every day. You can add many other ingredients to prevent boredom while following this program. In addition to the lettuce ingredients listed above, you can add any of the following:

+ pea shoots
+ alfalfa sprouts
+ broccoli sprouts

- onion sprouts
- clover sprouts
- mung bean sprouts
- chick peas
- kidney beans
- pinto beans
- lima beans
- Great Northern beans
- any other type of legume
- sliced strawberries
- apple slices
- orange slices
- grapefruit slices
- avocado
- green peppers
- red peppers
- yellow peppers
- finely chopped broccoli
- cucumber
- olives
- edible flowers
- grated carrots
- fresh peas
- grated cabbage
- freshly chopped parsley
- freshly chopped cilantro (coriander)
- any other freshly chopped herbs
- mushrooms (raw or cooked)
- green onion
- raspberries
- blueberries
- celery

Again, this list is by no means exhaustive. Let your imagination run wild to create delicious and nutritious gourmet salads.

You can eat from a variety of other lunch and dinner foods. I have included many recipes later in this book to give you some ideas. Follow the guidelines mentioned above. You can eat a large salad and a baked sweet potato, or a plate of brown rice pasta and vegetables. You could eat pasta salad or brown or wild rice in addition to your raw salad. You can eat a bean salad or lentil dahl. These are just some examples. See Chapter 13 for more ideas.

Eat an afternoon snack between meals. You can eat celery sticks with almond butter (see the recipes in Chapter 13), a piece of fruit, a handful of raw nuts and sunflower seeds, or drink a glass of soymilk. These are just some examples.

Be sure to drink at least eight to ten cups of pure water daily. Drink three cups of the water with eight drops of Cellfood® (see resources) per cup. You can squeeze lemon or lime into the remaining glasses of water. You can also deduct the herbal teas from your total water consumption.

Refrain from drinking water half an hour before meals or an hour after meals to avoid diluting your digestive enzymes. This allows your body to more completely digest your meals and helps to prevent bloating, allergies, or candida overgrowth in the intestines.

Now you have a good idea of the things to eat or not to eat, supplements to take, and exercise to do for all four weeks of *The 4-Week Ultimate Body Detox Plan*. To intensify cleansing of particular organs and organ systems, we will vary the program a bit, by adding specific herbs or nutrients for each of the four phases of the program.

You will cleanse the various detox organs and systems in a systematic approach, following four stages:

+ Phase 1: Cleansing the kidneys and bowels
+ Phase 2: Cleansing the lymphatic system (and this will help with cellulite as well)

- Phase 3: Cleansing the liver and gallbladder (and you will break down fatty deposits in your body too)
- Phase 4: Cleansing the blood, lungs, and skin

PHASE 1: CLEANSING THE KIDNEYS AND BOWELS

For Phase 1, drink the psyllium and pectin fibres mixed with pure cranberry juice and purified water, diluted 1:4 (one part cranberry juice to four parts water). I am referring to 100 percent pure cranberry juice, not cranberry cocktails or sweetened cranberry juice. Instead of water, you may wish to dilute cranberry juice with four parts of pure, unsweetened apple juice that contains no chemical additives or preservatives. This makes a much sweeter juice. You can blend this combination with a hand blender or coffee frother to make a smoother drink. It is imperative that you have at least one and a half cups of water or juice with this combination since the psyllium and pectin begin to swell once they get into your digestive tract. The water or apple juice helps to ensure there is adequate liquid to keep the mixture moving through your digestive tract. Wait at least ten minutes before eating anything else.

You may find that pure undiluted cranberry juice is quite expensive. Do not be alarmed by the price. You will actually be using a small amount at a time by diluting it with apple juice or water, which helps it to last.

Drink a second cup of the cranberry water blend during the day throughout Phase 1.

Eat an organic apple or two every day during Phase 1. Apples are healing for the kidneys and the intestinal tract, as they contain large amounts of water and a specific type of fibre called pectin. As I explained earlier, pectin binds to toxins and helps escort them out of the body in bowel movements.

Make a kidney tea blend of dried herbs: 1 part dandelion, 2 parts cleavers (an herb), 1 part buchu (an herb), and 1 part peppermint leaves. Mix and store in a glass container. Put one teaspoon of the dried herbal mixture in a tea ball or strainer. Pour 1 cup boiling water over it and infuse for ten minutes before drinking. If you want a sweeter drink, add two or three drops of liquid stevia, a natural herbal sweetener that is permitted while cleansing. Drink three cups of this herbal tea daily during Phase 1. Avoid this tea if you are diabetic. Alternatively, you can purchase dandelion leaf in capsules and take two capsules three times daily with meals during Phase 1.

PHASE 2: CLEANSING THE LYMPHATIC SYSTEM (AND CELLULITE)

Continue with the cranberry water during Phase 2. Again, drink one cup mixed with the psyllium and pectin and another cup on its own later in the day.

Make a lymphatic tea blend of dried herbs: 1 part echinacea, 2 parts cleavers, and 1 part peppermint leaves. Mix and store in a glass container. Put one teaspoon of the dried herbal mixture in a tea ball or strainer. Pour 1 cup boiling water over it and infuse for ten minutes before drinking. If you want a sweeter drink, add two or three drops of liquid stevia, a natural herbal sweetener that is permitted while cleansing. Drink three cups of this herbal tea daily during Phase 2. In addition, take astragalus in either tincture or capsule format. Follow the manufacturer's suggested dosage.

Continue to eat an organic apple daily and follow the dietary suggestions above.

PHASE 3: CLEANSING THE LIVER AND GALLBLADDER (AND FATTY DEPOSITS)

Instead of drinking the juice of half a lemon in a glass of water in the morning, increase the amount to the juice of a full lemon in a large glass of water first thing in the morning. You can also increase the amount of water if you prefer, to make it more palatable.

Take 4000 mg of lecithin daily. Take two digestive enzymes with every meal. In addition to the multivitamin you are already taking, add 2000 mg of vitamin C per day, divided into doses of 1000 mg at a time.

Make a liver-gallbladder tea blend of dried herbs: 1 part dandelion root, 1 part ginger root, 1 part turmeric, and 1 part chicory. Mix and store in a glass container. In a small saucepan, mix four teaspoons of the dried herbal mixture in four cups of water. Bring to a boil. Simmer for twenty minutes, covered. Drink one cup, three times per day. Refrigerate the remainder until you are ready to drink it. Sweeten with stevia if you prefer.

In addition, take a milk thistle seed supplement in capsule form. Take two 250 mg capsules at a time, three times a day with meals. The supplement should be a standardized 80 percent extract of *Silybum marianum*.

PHASE 4: CLEANSING THE BLOOD, LUNGS, AND SKIN

Drink a quarter cup of pure aloe vera juice, diluted in water if you prefer, after your lemon water in the morning. Drink an additional quarter cup of aloe vera juice in the afternoon. Avoid using "aloes" or "aloe latex" since these versions can be too harsh for the body. Avoid aloe juice if you are pregnant.

You should have been taking a green food supplement during the last several weeks. Double the amount of green food supplement you are taking during Phase 4. The additional chlorophyll (green colour naturally found in plants) will assist with blood purification.

If you have a juicer, drink the skin cleansing juice (listed in Chapter 13) daily.

Supplement with 400 IU of a high-quality vitamin E capsule daily. Ideally, it should be a mixed tocopherol blend of gamma tocopherol, delta tocopherol, and beta tocopherol.

Make a blood-lungs-skin cleansing tea blend of dried herbs: 1 part coltsfoot, 1 part comfrey, and 1 part horehound. Mix and store in a glass container. Put one teaspoon of the dried herbal mixture in a tea ball or strainer. Pour 1 cup boiling water over it and infuse for ten minutes before drinking. If you want a sweeter drink, add several drops of liquid stevia. Drink three cups of this herbal tea daily during Phase 4.

This program is designed to be flexible. After each phase, take the brief quizzes listed in the following chapters to help you determine whether the allotted one-week phase is sufficient for you or if you might benefit from staying at one phase for a longer period before moving to the next phase. For example, if after one week of cleansing the lymphatic system in Phase 2 of *The 4-Week Ultimate Body Detox Plan*, you still have cellulite that you would like to target, you can stay in Phase 2 for a longer period before moving to Phase 3: Cleansing the Liver and Gallbladder (and Fat Deposits). You can also incorporate the cleansing suggestions such as the herbs and energy medicine techniques suggested in Chapter 9 into the four-week detox plan.

While the program has been designed for a four-week period, I recognize that everyone is different and therefore has different needs. This approach allows you the flexibility to customize the program for optimum results.

Bear in mind that you will be cleansing all the body's detoxification systems to some degree during all phases of the program; however, your efforts will be greatly targeted to allow deeper and more extensive cleansing. For example, you will not suddenly stop cleansing the kidneys and bowels once you leave Phase 1. That will continue, just to a lesser degree, while you are cleansing the lymph system, liver and gallbladder, blood, lungs, and skin during the following phases.

Cleansing your body's many detoxification organs will require some effort, but the rewards will be worth it. Perseverance is critical.

After you get started forming new habits, your body will actually begin to crave healthy fuel. Remember, you are trying to undo years of poor eating habits that take some effort to change. A positive attitude will make sticking to the program much easier.

Essential Grocery List

Green food supplement

Cellfood®

High-quality full-spectrum enzyme (should ideally contain amylase, protease, lipase, cellulase, peptidase, maltase, lactase, and invertase)

High-quality multivitamin and multimineral

Flora supplement (should contain *Lactobacillus acidophilus* and *Bifidobacterium*)

Pectin

Psyllium husks/hulls

Pure water

Stevia, unpasteurized honey, or 100% pure maple syrup (for use in moderation only)

Celtic sea salt (for use in moderation only)

Lemons

Plenty of fresh fruits and vegetables (preferably organic)

In this chapter you learned
+ How to decrease your exposure to toxins in your foods and beverages
+ How to effectively eliminate toxic buildup in all of your body's detoxification organs
+ The best order in which to cleanse your body's detoxification organs

References

1. Helen Foster, *Detox Solutions* (London: Octopus Publishing Group Ltd., 2004), p. 17.

2. Foster, *Detox Solutions*, p. 17.

3. Foster, *Detox Solutions*, p. 18.

4. Kathleen Barnes, "The Little Fiber Pill That Can Detox Your Whole Body," *Woman's World*, April 27, 2004, p. 24.

CHAPTER 6

Power-Packed Detoxification

It is better to light a candle than to curse the darkness.
The Christophers

In this chapter you will learn
+ Ways to increase the benefits of detoxification
+ A skin brushing technique that improves the flow of your lymphatic system
+ A rebound workout that stimulates lymphatic system flow and improves circulation
+ How to incorporate a simple hydrotherapy technique into your detox plan to improve circulation;
+ A simple lymph-stimulating bath and lymphatic massage
+ How to make simple and effective herbal teas for cleansing
+ Acupressure techniques to assist with cleansing
+ Energy balancing techniques that assist with cleansing

There are many wonderful techniques that you can incorporate into *The 4-Week Ultimate Body Detox Plan*, that not only assist your body with detoxification, but also feel great. Using simple techniques such as skin brushing, rebounding, hydrotherapy, lymph stimulating baths, lymphatic massage, acupressure, and an energy medicine technique, you will probably feel more like you are at a spa than on a detox program.

Some of the techniques are incorporated throughout *The 4-Week Ultimate Body Detox Plan*, while others are suitable for specific phases. If you feel you would benefit from any of these techniques, feel free to include them as well. At the end of each therapy type, I have listed its main focus for the purpose of detoxification as Phases 1, 2, 3, and 4; Phase 1; Phase 2; Phase 3; Phase 4; or Optional for Phase 1; Optional for Phase 2; Optional for Phase 3; and Optional for Phase 4.

SKIN BRUSHING

Skin brushing is a simple technique that improves circulation and lymphatic flow. It is part of the whole *4-Week Ultimate Body Detox Plan* because it is such a great way to assist your body with toxin elimination. Most health food stores carry natural-bristle brushes. Ideally, you will want one with a handle with medium to firm bristles. To skin brush:

+ First, massage below your collarbone and on left and right sides of the groin area on your upper legs using firm finger pressure.
+ Then, brush the soles of your feet in a circular motion moving upward over your legs using the natural-bristle brush. Brush over your stomach and buttocks to your waist, continuing to use a circular motion.
+ Continue to brush in a circular motion over the palms of your hands.

- Using long, upward strokes, brush over the rest of your hands and arms.
- Brush from your neck to shoulders, down your chest or breasts and down your back.

Perform this simple exercise daily before showering or bathing. Once you are familiar with it, it takes only a minute or two. Do not skin-brush before bed since it can be energizing to your body and may prevent restful sleep.

I recommend skin brushing throughout *The 4-Week Ultimate Body Detox Plan*, but you may wish to continue if you have problems with your circulation, such as cold hands and feet, or if your lymphatic system is sluggish. You will learn how to tell if your lymphatic system is sluggish in Chapter 9. **Phases 1, 2, 3, and 4**

REBOUND WORKOUT
- Walk-bounce at an easy pace for 5 minutes.
- Flat-bounce with feet about 1 foot apart for 5 minutes.
- March-bounce with swinging arms for 3 minutes.
- Walk-bounce for 5 minutes.
- Do this five times a week, eventually adding five more minutes of march-bouncing and "lymph activator" bouncing (straight legs, feet come about three inches off mat).

I recommend rebounding daily throughout *The 4-Week Ultimate Body Detox Plan* and continuing it to maintain lymphatic system cleansing.
Phase 2

HYDROTHERAPY
Alternating hot and cold showers stimulates lymphatic circulation. One way to do this is to jump into a hot shower for several minutes

(as hot as is still comfortable), then to change the temperature to be cold for another several minutes (if you can stand it that long). Repeat this hot and cold pattern at least one more time each. The heat dilates the blood vessels and the cold causes them to contract. Avoid this type of therapy if you have heart or blood pressure problems or if you are pregnant. Consult a holistically minded physician if you are unsure whether this hydrotherapy treatment is suitable for you.

This hydrotherapy treatment is best used during Phase 2, but you may wish to continue using it throughout *The 4-Week Ultimate Body Detox Plan* or afterward to continue cleansing your lymphatic system.

Optional for Phases 2 and 4

LYMPH-STIMULATING BATH

I am still amazed when I consider a hot bath as therapy for any health issue. To me the pleasures of a warm bath combined with decadent aromatherapy oils just feel s-o-o-o-o good that I tend to forget its therapeutic properties. A blend of specific aromatherapy oils that stimulate the lymphatic system can be used in the bath for this purpose. Into a small container, put three drops of each of the following: pure geranium, juniper, and black pepper oils; blend with one tablespoon of oil such as grapeseed, apricot kernel, or almond oil (referred to as carrier oils). Add to a bath. Alternatively, if you have only one of the above oils available, you can add nine drops of it to the carrier oil of your choice and add it to your bath.

Simply dunk your body for twenty minutes or so, lie back, relax, and let the healing power of water and plant oils work their magic.

The lymph-stimulating bath is most suited for lymphatic cleansing (Phase 2 of this program) but you can continue using it several times per week if you need additional lymphatic system cleansing.

Optional for Phase 2

LYMPHATIC MASSAGE

You can improve the flow of your lymphatic system by massaging your body. Use three drops of each of the following essential oils: geranium, juniper, and black pepper; dilute them in three tablespoons of another oil (this oil is often called a carrier oil). You can use any of the following carrier oils: grapeseed, apricot kernel, or almond oil.

Massage your arms and legs using long upward strokes, moving toward your heart.

Lymphatic massage is recommended during Phase 2 of this program, but you can continue using it for lymphatic system cleansing and maintenance of lymphatic system health.
Optional for Phases 2 and 4

CLEANSING HERBAL TEAS

In the coming chapters you will learn about many cleansing herbs for the various detoxification systems. I will provide suggestions on how to best incorporate the herbs into the detox plan. Herbs are Nature's medicines and should be treated as such. Over 80 percent of our current pharmaceutical drugs are based on substances originally found in herbs. In the herbs, the substances are natural. In the pharmaceutical drugs, the active ingredients in plants are synthesized to enable manufacturers to patent the "new" synthetic ingredient and to profit from it. The human body responds best to the medicines that Nature intended for it—the natural ones found in herbs.

Having been in the holistic health industry for over seventeen years, I have developed an enormous pet peeve. Here it is: It drives me crazy to hear people say that they don't believe in herbs. What on earth is that supposed to mean? As someone who has a massive health library (just ask the builder of my home who built me wall-to-wall bookshelves that still didn't hold all my books) that cites the thousands, yes thousands, of scientific studies that *prove* the medicinal properties of herbs, it amazes me how ignorant some people actually choose to remain.

Herbal medicine is quite safe when used appropriately. Many people, the media included, blame herbs when there is a drug-herb interaction. Herbs are medicines and drugs are medicines. Of course they will interact. It is imperative that you consult with a skilled herbalist or a pharmacist who is knowledgeable about herbs (a rare find) before combining them. Also, avoid taking larger amounts of the herbs suggested. The "more is better" mentality does not apply to herbs and, similar to medication, can cause toxic reactions.

If you are pregnant or nursing or have any serious health concerns, you should contact your holistic health-care professional before taking any herbal remedies.

A significant body of evidence demonstrates the effectiveness of hundreds of different herbs for cleansing and rebuilding the body. Every day, the list of scientific evidence of the healing power of herbs grows.

You can typically find dried herbs or herbal preparations known as tinctures at your local health food store. Tinctures are concentrated extracts of herbs, usually in an alcohol base. The alcohol assists with extracting the medicinal properties of the plants and acts as a natural preservative for the herbal preparation. The amount of alcohol you will consume while taking these remedies is quite small and therefore is not a health concern for most people; however, if you cannot tolerate any herbal preparations in an alcohol base, you can frequently find herbal extracts in a vegetable glycerine base as well.

You can also make herbal teas from the herbs mentioned in the coming chapters. You can purchase the dried, loose herbs at your local health food store and make herbal teas. It is important to understand that there are two different types of herbal teas: infusions and decoctions.

An infusion is made in the same way you would make black or green tea using loose-leaf tea. Use the amount of dried herb suggested in the following chapters; place it into a tea ball or strainer and pour one cup of boiling water over it. Let it sit for five to ten minutes. Strain and drink. Alternatively, you can triple the amount of herb suggested and pour three cups of boiling water over it to make enough for the day. Then drink one cup at a time, three times per day (or the amount suggested under the particular herb description).

Some herbs are best made into decoctions to help extract their medicinal properties. Again, measure the amount of dried herb suggested, pour one cup of water over it (or triple the dried herb and use three cups of water for ease throughout the day) into a pot. Bring the mixture to a boil and allow it to boil for ten minutes. Strain and drink (or, if tripling the recipe, divide into three equal doses).

Herbal teas are recommended for each of the four phases of *The 4 Week Ultimate Body Detox Program.* They help your body handle toxins more effectively, while strengthening the body's detox organs. They should be included in every phase of your detoxification program.

ACUPRESSURE FOR DETOXIFICATION

Imagine being struck by an arrow in an ancient battle, then recovering from the wound, only to discover that your lifelong chest pains and breathing difficulties had disappeared. That is the legend behind the formation of acupuncture. Wounded soldiers were believed to have experienced the sudden healing of afflictions (that existed prior to battle) along with the recovery of the arrow wound.

Tradition also states that acupuncture formed out of a dialogue between the Chinese ruler Huang Di (the "Yellow Emperor") and his prime minister, Chi Po. No one knows exactly how this ancient healing art was first discovered, but it has stood the test of time, existing for ten thousand years because it is remarkably effective for healing and pain reduction. Slight variations of it developed independently in China and India and among the ancient Aztecs. Compare this lengthy history to "modern medicine," which has been around for only a hundred years or so.

Thousands of research studies have proven the healing effects of needling the body in specific locations known as points or acupoints, but millions of people have experienced the proof that acupuncture works just by witnessing improvements in their symptoms. For those in need of scientific proof, engineers developed instruments called acupunctuscopes that prove the existence of the acupuncture points by reading the electrical frequency on the surface of the skin. Changes in electrical frequency occur in the exact location of the points on the body based on ancient texts and drawings.

These points exist in the body in connected lines known as meridians or channels. While many studies had proved the existence of the acupuncture points, until recently scientists still doubted that they were connected. Over a decade ago, French scientists went to work to prove or disprove the meridian theory. Taking two groups of people, they injected them with radioactive dye. One group was injected with dye in the exact location of the acupuncture points. Participants in the other group were injected in bogus points. The movement of the dye was monitored. Researchers were shocked to discover that where the dye had been injected into real acupuncture points, it flowed in lines in the positions of the meridians recorded by the Chinese millennia ago. Where the dye was injected into bogus points, the dye merely dispersed, without following any lines at all. Other studies have also confirmed the existence of meridians in the body.

Even the World Health Organization endorses acupuncture by publishing a list of dozens of illnesses that acupuncture effectively treats, including headaches and migraines; osteoarthritis, bursitis, tendonitis, sciatica, and other musculoskeletal disorders; neurological disorders; and countless others.

Essentially, the meridians are energy pathways in the body that, when flowing properly, ensure health and vitality. However, when a blockage occurs (which can be caused by any number of things including stress, physical injuries, emotional traumas, allergies, and poor nutrition) the flow of energy is disrupted and this disruption can cause a multitude of symptoms including pain, inflammation and virtually any health problem. Energy meridians are similar to a river. If a tree falls in the river, it may disrupt the flow of water through the river and may even affect any tributaries that get their flow of water from the river. A blockage is comparable to the tree, disrupting the proper energy flow throughout the body.

The acupoints are locations along the energy lines where the energy surfaces in the body. These are the locations that the Chinese (and other cultures) documented over five thousand years ago, and whose existence recent research has confirmed. These points, with their higher electrical frequency, respond very well to touch applied in the form of pressure or massage.

In China, acupuncture is practised widely in hospitals and medical clinics. In the West, however, it has taken longer to catch on. Perhaps this is due to our experiences with needles, which we associate with large, thick instruments used for drawing blood or delivering vaccinations—the kind that make you jump out of your chair from discomfort or fear. Unlike these needles, acupuncture needles are quite fine, much thinner than a pin, in fact.

How can this knowledge help you? You can use it to supercharge your cleansing efforts by applying a form of modified acupuncture known as acupressure on yourself. Acupressure uses simple finger pressure to alleviate blockages in the body, without the use of needles. Both techniques are effective.

I have included specific acupressure for helping to cleanse and improve the functioning of your detox organs, which you will find in the appropriate chapters. For example, in Chapter 8, you will learn kidney acupressure points and in Chapter 10, you will explore acupressure for improving liver and gallbladder function.

Because the basic technique is the same and only the points vary, I am including it here. Although there are hundreds of acupressure points on the body, I will be including only the main ones for improving detox functions. The points are named after the organ meridian on which they appear. For example, Kidney 1, also referred to as K 1, is the first point of the Kidney meridian. Stomach 36 (St 36) is the thirty-sixth point along the Stomach meridian.

While proponents of acupressure often espouse specific approaches to pressing or rubbing the points, you can get great results from doing what feels right for you and not getting caught up in theory. You can either firmly hold the points or rub them in small clockwise circles, whichever feels best to you. I find that firmly holding the points typically gives better results.

I recommend that you not use massage oils or lotions when rubbing the points, as these will make your skin too slippery to hold the point for any length of time. In fact, you can be fully clothed while doing acupressure, making it easy to do anywhere. Some of the points are easily accessible and allow you to rub them on a bus ride or in the car (as a passenger, of course), or while watching television. If it is difficult for you to use your thumb or fingers to rub the points, you can also use your knuckle.

Avoid getting stressed about whether you're finding the point precisely. Sometimes, there will be some discomfort at the site of the point, while other times there won't be any noticeable sensation.

The points we will be using are located on both sides of the body. I recommend holding the points on both sides of the body (at the same time if you prefer) for best results.

When trying to locate an acupressure point, a general rule of thumb is if you find a point on your body that feels sore, apply firm pressure. You may have discovered an energy blockage. Pressing on the area will help to disperse any blockages you might have. Do not be overly aggressive while pressing the area or you may cause bruising. At the same time, apply enough pressure to really feel the acupressure.[1]

If you are pregnant or have any serious health concerns, consult a qualified acupuncturist before proceeding. Acupressure is quite safe with no side effects that I am aware of. If you are pregnant, you can simply avoid the following points: Large Intestine (LI 4), Stomach 36 (St 36), Spleen 6 (Sp6), Kidney 3 (K3), Urinary Bladder 36 (UB36), and avoid massaging the abdomen. Avoid using acupressure during the first and last trimester of pregnancy as well.

Specific acupressure techniques are listed in Chapters 8, 10, and 11, depending on their use for cleansing. Use them during the corresponding phase of the program. For example, in Phase 1, you can incorporate the acupressure techniques listed in Chapter 8, "Targeting Your Kidneys and Intestines." You may wish to continue using the acupressure to maintain your cleansing results after you are finished *The 4-Week Ultimate Body Detox Plan*. (Specific exercises appear under their respective phases.)

ENERGY BALANCING TECHNIQUES FOR CLEANSING

As you learned from the studies mentioned regarding acupressure, energy exists in our body. Many other studies confirm this. Albert Einstein was one of the leading scientists who furthered our knowledge of energy when he created the mathematical equation, $E=mc^2$. Although it is not essential to our cleansing program that you understand the meaning of this equation, suffice it to say that the "E" stands for "energy," and Einstein said matter and energy are two different forms of the same thing.

Einstein was not the first to believe in the existence of energy. Throughout many cultures, the concept of a subtle force that flows through and around the body is not new. In China, the existence of energy is the foundation for acupuncture, which we now know to have existed for approximately ten thousand years. In the yogic tradition of India and Tibet, people have long understood the concept of energy, which they call *prana*. The Jewish Kabbalistic tradition refers to energy as *yesod*. In the Christian faith, energy is often called The Holy Spirit. The Lakota tribe of the First Peoples of North America called energy *wakan*. The Iroquois tribe refers to this subtle, yet powerful force as *orenda*.

Although most people cannot see energy, it nevertheless exists. It is comparable to electricity. We can see the wires and the end result of its existence, light or heat, but we cannot see electricity itself. The same is true of nuclear power. We do not see it, but we see the results, and we certainly see those results when things go wrong. Most people may not be able to see energy, but without its existence life would cease.

Einstein found that everything in the world is made up of energy, regardless of whether we are referring to animate or inanimate objects, human or non-human, living or supposedly non-living beings. Everything radiates energy. Energy flows through, between, and around every cell in your body. It therefore flows through every organ and organ system. We must help ensure a balanced flow of energy throughout the body to ensure properly functioning organs and organ systems.

The basic premise of energy medicine, the body of knowledge that manipulates energy for healing purposes, great health, and disease prevention, is that matter follows energy. Or, as Donna Eden and David Feinstein, two of the foremost energy medicine practitioners, state in their book *Energy Medicine*, "When your energies are vibrant, so is your body."[2] Since healthy energies *precede* great health, it is imperative that any good detox program incorporate energy balancing techniques.

I asked Donna and David to recommend some powerful energy medicine techniques, which they describe in their aptly named book *Energy Medicine*, for the purpose of cleansing the body and its various detox organs.[3] Based on their suggestions, I have included numerous energy medicine techniques in Chapters 7 through 11, choosing the best technique for particular cleansing purposes. They will improve the flow of energy to, through, and around the organs to help them cleanse and rebuild.

Phases 1, 2, 3, and 4 (Specific exercises appear under their respective phases [Chapters 8 to 11].)

> In this chapter you learned
> - You can increase your body's ability to cleanse toxins and emotions using simple techniques that feel great
> - You can assist your lymphatic system to eliminate toxins using skin brushing, rebounding, hydrotherapy, a lymph-stimulating bath, lymphatic massage, and energy balancing techniques
> - You can assist with cleansing your blood using skin brushing, rebounding, hydrotherapy, and lymphatic massage
> - You can use acupressure techniques (which you will learn in the following chapters) to help cleanse your urinary and intestinal tracts, liver and gallbladder, lungs and skin
> - You can use various energy balancing techniques (which you will learn in the following chapters) to cleanse your urinary and intestinal tracts, lymphatic system, liver and gallbladder, blood, lungs, and skin

References

1. Some of this material previously appeared in Michelle Schoffro Cook, *Healing Injuries the Natural Way* (Toronto: Your Health Press, 2004).

2. Donna Eden and David Feinstein, *Energy Medicine* (New York: Jeremy P. Tarcher/Penguin, 1998), p. 17.

3. The energy medicine techniques in this book are reproduced with the permission of Donna Eden and David Feinstein. For additional information on these or other energy techniques, I suggest referring to their book, *Energy Medicine.* (see resources)

CHAPTER 7

Emotional Detox Strategies

The little space within the heart is as great as the vast universe.
The heavens and the earth are there, and the sun and the moon and
the stars. Fire and lightning and winds are there, and all that
now is and all that is not.
Upanishads

In this chapter you will learn
- The 10 Emotional Detox Principles
- Simple meditation exercises that you can use when you need an instant pick-me-up or an immediate release of tension, at home, work, or almost anywhere
- Easy yoga exercises
- Ancient Chinese qigong exercises
- The benefits of meditating and energy exercises; and
- The effects of toxic people in our lives and suggestions for dealing with them

One of the most important elements of great health is a positive attitude. Research confirms that there is a strong mind-body link that can positively or negatively affect health, healing, and the ability to ward off or fight disease.

Researchers have developed an Optimism-Pessimism (PSM) scale in a study referred to as the Minnesota Multiphasic Personality Inventory (MMPI). This study showed that people with a pessimistic attitude have poorer health, are prone to depression, are more frequent users of medical and mental health-care systems, exhibit more mental decline as they age, and have impaired immune functions and a shorter survival rate than optimists.[1]

Stressful emotions create damaging hormones and toxins in the body. The adrenal glands, the body's main "stress" glands, secrete hormones to help us deal with short-term stresses. However, in our modern times, many people live under constant stress. The body does not differentiate between life-threatening stresses, such as being chased by a sabre-toothed tiger, which our distant ancestors might have experienced thousands of years ago, and our current stresses, such as job stress, relationship difficulties, or money worries. It is important that we learn mechanisms to release stress buildup and improve our abilities to cope with stress.

This reminds me of work I did in the international trade realm. North American clients would inevitably claim that everything was urgent. They would hire my services as a consultant, expecting me to make up for their time delays by working day and night. Some of the European clients I worked with would also claim that their project was urgent, while allowing weeks for its completion. Their approach was far more relaxed and reasonable.

We have a tendency to overestimate the urgency of our work and live somewhat myopic lives at times, believing that virtually all our experiences are highly stressful. I felt that way at one time and still occasionally get sucked into this unrealistic pattern. However, when I was very ill and questioned whether I would continue living, my view of stress changed substantially. Lying on my bed, unable to *do* anything, I had to learn to love myself, not for what I was able to do or for any accomplishments or achievements, but for who I am. It was at that time that I realized I had lived my whole life to that point believing that I was the sum of my successes and failures. I felt like an empty shell of a person. I also came to learn that stress is really a figment of our imaginations. Life is only as stressful as we choose to let it be. I know there will be people who choose to become angered by this statement.

We are the only directors of our lives. We are the only ones who choose our responses. We can choose to make the most of our life experiences or not, depending on our outlook on life. As a stress release mechanism, I started to ask myself, "Will this matter at the end of my life? Or even in a year?" If the answer was no, then I would take some deep breaths, do the energy exercise described later in this chapter, and get on with my day.

We know that stress affects our hormones, which can be damaging to our health over the long term. Research also suggests that emotions can become stored at the cellular level. This could be part of the reason why we can become stuck in the traumas we endure. Other studies demonstrate that stress can cause blockages in our energy systems.

To fully detoxify, it is essential to consider stress and our emotions and follow an emotional detox program to help rid our bodies and minds of stress buildup. Before you can benefit from some of the emotional detoxification techniques I am about to share with you, it is important to recognize that emotions play a huge role in your physical health. Although disease may have roots in the physical body, in my opinion, it just as often has emotional roots.

Research in a field of study known as psychoneuroimmunology found that *every* part of our immune system is linked to the brain. Researchers discovered that every thought, experience, and emotion sends messages to the immune system, either strengthening or impairing its functioning. Emotions such as happiness, optimism, and joy boost the immune system, while pessimism and depression are linked to an increased risk of cancer.[2]

In another long-term study of older men, scientists found that men who had high levels of optimism had a 45 percent lower risk of angina pectoris, non-fatal heart attack, and coronary heart disease-related death, than men who were less optimistic. Other research shows that worry and anger are associated with an increased risk of cardiovascular disease.[3]

To prevent emotional stress from affecting your overall health and well-being, it is important to recognize how your attitude or approach to life may affect your health. There are ten major Emotional Detox Principles that can help with this.

EMOTIONAL DETOX PRINCIPLE 1: YOU ARE THE DIRECTOR OF YOUR LIFE

Either this is an empowering principle or it can feel like a tonne of bricks hitting you, depending on where you are in life. We've all had moments of being victimized by our circumstances but the people who make significant life improvements are those who refuse to fall prey to self-pity. If you look around your life and do not like what you see, you can choose to feel sorry for yourself or you can recognize that somewhere along the way in creating your life, you may have got off track. We all do sometimes. To truly direct your life in the way you want to go, you have to take full responsibility as the Director—with all the feelings of success and failure that accompany that role.

EMOTIONAL DETOX PRINCIPLE 2: REAL LIFE CHANGES REQUIRE SHIFTS IN ATTITUDE

You may have heard the adage "If you always do what you've always done, you'll always get what you've always got." If you are content with everything in your life, then continue what you always do, but if you want to change your life you need to change your attitude and the things you are doing. Proust said, "The real voyage of discovery consists not in seeing new landscapes but in having new eyes." Shift your view to be one that is positive, and you'll be amazed at the discoveries you make along the way. A positive outlook makes a tremendous difference and can help you to totally transform your existing life into the life of your dreams.

EMOTIONAL DETOX PRINCIPLE 3: BE HONEST WITH YOURSELF

If you don't like something in your life, have the courage to be honest with yourself. This is more difficult than it seems sometimes. We often delude ourselves into accepting aspects of our life so we will not have to put in the effort to make changes. Honesty is an integral part of remaking your life into the life you would like to have.

EMOTIONAL DETOX PRINCIPLE 4: NURTURE AND RESPECT YOURSELF

The Upanishads may have stated this principle best: "The little space within the heart is as great as the vast universe. The heavens and the earth are there, and the sun and the moon and the stars. Fire and lightning and winds are there, and all that now is and all that is not." You are greatness personified. Treat your body, mind, and spirit with the respect they deserve. If you love yourself, don't feed your body junk, don't accept emotionally or physically abusive treatment, don't accept less than you deserve.

EMOTIONAL DETOX PRINCIPLE 5: TODAY'S THOUGHTS AND ACTIONS CREATE TOMORROW'S REALITY

I recently asked one of my clients, "Who is thinking the thoughts of uncertainty, questioning whether you will ever recover from your illness?" Her response is obvious—she is the only thinker in her mind. While there may be plenty of social conditioning that affects us, we are the only ones who can choose to accept thoughts and ideas as part of our reality. You are the only thinker of your thoughts. Those thoughts will create your reality. If you don't like the reality your thoughts are creating, change your thoughts.

I am still amazed at the number of people, even medical doctors, who tell me, "I don't believe that thoughts or emotions play a role in a person's health." The research that proves this connection is voluminous. This is not about believing. This is *proven*. Saying something like that is almost like saying, "I don't believe in electricity because I can't see it." You can still reap the beneficial effects of electricity without having an understanding of its inner workings.

You become what you think and feel. Research even shows that thinking and feeling compassionate thoughts produce measurable changes in the electrical activity of the heart.[4]

A recent study by Dr. Suzanne Segerstrom at the University of Kentucky on the role of stress and the immune system in first-year law students found that those students who remained optimistic under stress had more helper T cells and more effective killer T cells (two indications of a strong immune system) than pessimistic students.

Want to feel great? Start thinking positive thoughts and expressing positive emotions.

EMOTIONAL DETOX PRINCIPLE 6: CELEBRATE SUCCESS

Celebrate every success along your journey, no matter how small. A friend of mine laughed at me because every time I had a seemingly small success in my life, I would celebrate, not with decadence and overindulgence, but with small things that I enjoyed. I would take a moment out of my day to enjoy some soy chai (Indian spiced tea), cook up my favourite healthy dinner (yes, healthy dinners can taste great too), have a long aromatherapy bath, or take a break from my day to share my success with my husband (my life's best cheering section). Choose small things that you enjoy to celebrate every success along your journey. Of course, it is important to choose things that are healthful. Going out for beers with the guys to celebrate every small success would violate Principle 4: Nurture and *Respect* Yourself.

Also, it is important to celebrate other people's successes. If you choose to belittle people or diminish the success of others, then you violate a significant Emotional Detox Principle and you will see limited success in your own life. Examine your life for areas where there may be hidden cynicism toward success. For example, many people believe that rich people are not good people, that they are snobs. That may be true of some rich people, but I have also met poor people who are snobs. Celebrate the success of others, including financial success.

EMOTIONAL DETOX PRINCIPLE 7: SURROUND YOURSELF WITH SUPPORTIVE AND POSITIVE PEOPLE

Nobody needs someone kicking them down every time their life starts to improve, or worse, telling them, "I told you so" every time they hit an obstacle along the road to the life of their dreams. Life can be like a garden. If you don't weed it regularly, the weeds will overgrow the plants and flowers you're trying to nurture. The same is true of people. While everyone has potential to nurture the greatness within him- or herself, not everyone chooses to do that. Some people are downright negative or nasty. You only have so much time in a day. Choose to spend that time with people who are positive and support you on your journey.

EMOTIONAL DETOX PRINCIPLE 8: YOU GET WHAT YOU GIVE OUT

Someone once remarked while I was out hiking that everyone I encountered on the paths smiled at me. That person then realized that I was smiling at the people I met. They were smiling back. I found that people are far friendlier when you are friendly to them. If you're always miserable, negative, or just barely tolerable, you will find that life hands you miserable, negative, or just barely tolerable experiences. Put on a smile and the world smiles back at you. Research even shows that you can trick your brain into thinking you are happy by smiling and telling yourself that you are. Before you know it, you are happy.

EMOTIONAL DETOX PRINCIPLE 9: SHARE YOUR SUCCESS WITH OTHERS

Share your good fortune with others, by sharing the principles that helped you along your journey, by taking the time to help people in need, and by contributing to worthy causes. We are intricately connected with every other living being on this planet, and with Mother Nature. By sharing our success, it comes back to us many times over. I would like to share Gandhi's Prayer for Peace to help you on your journey: "I offer you peace. I offer you love. I offer you friendship. I see your beauty. I hear your need. I feel your feelings. My wisdom flows from the Highest Source. I salute that Source in you. Let us work together for unity and love."

EMOTIONAL DETOX PRINCIPLE 10: KEEP ON TRUCKING

There is a common expression among professional writers that the difference between success and failure as a writer has nothing to do with skill and everything to do with persistence. While skill is necessary in life, persistence to transform your life will be one of the greatest factors in your success.

Henry David Thoreau wrote, "Go confidently in the direction of your dreams. Live the life you've imagined." I encourage you to go confidently in the direction of your dreams. By doing so, you have a much better chance to live a fulfilling and happy life.

Now I would like to share with you some powerful emotional detox techniques to help you emotionally and energetically cleanse.

EMOTIONAL DETOX TECHNIQUES

There are many excellent emotional detox techniques—enough to make up a book-length work on their own. I have selected only a few, but they are ones I have had tremendous success with, for myself and for my clients. You do not need to perform all the emotional detox techniques. Simply choose the one or ones that most appeal to you and stick with them throughout the four weeks of detoxification.

One thing I have witnessed countless times is that people who choose to follow only the nutritional and herbal suggestions will often re-experience old traumas or emotions as part of their cleansing efforts. This is natural and a positive experience. I believe that the body uses detoxification as a means to emotionally cleanse as well. Incorporating emotional cleansing techniques into the overall detox program produces the best results. You will have tools at your disposal to help lessen the discomfort of painful emotions. You will also be better able to eliminate old traumas permanently, instead of pushing them back down, only to see them resurface later.

Some of the techniques I have included are keeping a detox journal, meditation, breathing exercises, energy exercises, and Bach flower therapy. After reading about and trying the various techniques, choose the one or ones that feel best for you. Keep in mind that sometimes we avoid the very things we would most benefit from. Meditation is a perfect example. Many people avoid quietening their minds through meditation because they fear the feelings that exist when their mental chatter stops. If that sounds like you, I urge you to begin to meditate.

Keep a Detox Journal

Now that you've learned the Emotional Detox Principles, it is time to start incorporating them into your detox program. During the next four weeks, begin to keep a Detox Journal. Take a few minutes every day to make note of your emotions as they arise. A common experience I hear from clients who undertake my detox programs is that they often gain a new perspective on old problems that have been weighing them down. By keeping a Detox Journal you will better enable your body to let go of troubling thoughts and emotions to live a more positive life.

What exactly are you going to write in this journal? Write about your physical, mental, and emotional experiences throughout cleansing. Write about any issues you are currently facing or problems that do not seem to be resolved. Write about your dreams, hopes, fear, doubts, and what you want from your life. This is your detox journal. No one will be grading it so you can write whatever is on your mind.

Avoid censoring the thoughts and feelings that come to you as you write in your journal. Allow your feelings to flow naturally without criticism or judgements. If you feel angry, write it down. If you feel sadness or grief, write it down. If you feel joy, write it down. Write exactly how you feel. By choosing this emotional cleansing practice, many people discover how removed they are from their true feelings. By keeping busy in a fast-paced life, it is easy to lose track of our true feelings. Reconnect to them by journalling.

Qigong Ancient Breathing Technique

The following emotional detox technique is a powerful ancient breathing exercise that can be found in ancient Chinese teachings called qigong (pronounced "chee-gung"). It will help improve your energy, increase your concentration, and release stress. Decreasing stress helps your body focus on existing toxins, instead of overburdening it with stress hormones the existing toxins.

Stand with your feet shoulder-width apart. Bend your knees slightly. Let your arms fall limp at your sides. Lower your shoulders to relax any tension. Tuck in your chin and pull your head back, keeping it in alignment with your spine. Close your eyes, rest your tongue on the roof of your mouth, and take a deep breath through your nose, expanding your belly as you inhale. When you inhale, do not force the breath—just let it gradually become deeper and deeper. With every inhalation, imagine energy from the earth rising up from the soles

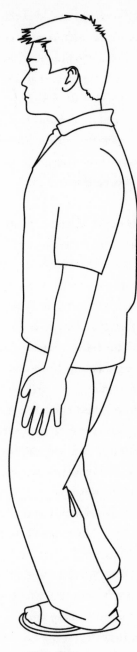

Figure 7.1 Qigong posture

of your feet and up the front of your body, purifying your body as it moves. Then with every exhalation through your nose, visualize the energy flowing down the back of your body, still purifying your whole body as it traverses. Visualize the stale energy full of toxins returning to the earth to be purified. Breathe in fresh energy from the earth and continue as before for at least five minutes.

Perform this simple breathing exercise throughout your day whenever you need energy, or to relax, or just to feel greater peace in your life.

There are many forms of qigong that include diverse postures and movements. This simple exercise is a good point of departure should you wish to delve further into this ancient practice.

Xiu Lian Body Power Technique[5]

Dr. Zhi Gang Sha describes a technique for cleansing and healing in his book *Power Healing*. The practice of Xiu Lian (pronounced "shoo lee-en") has existed in Chinese culture for the last five thousand years. According to Dr. Sha, "Xiu means to purify your heart, mind, and soul. It means having love, care, compassion, sincerity, honesty, generosity, integrity, unselfishness, and discipline. It also means accumulating virtue and giving service to people and society. Lian means to practice all of these things in your daily life, in your actions, behaviours, and thoughts."

He explains how to perform this simple, yet powerful technique: "Sit comfortably with your back straight, but not leaning against anything. Keep both feet on the floor. Relax. Place your hands in front of your chest. Gently touch the heels of your hands together, gently touch your thumbs together, and gently touch your little fingers together. Open your hands and fingers as though you were holding a beautiful lotus flower. Relax and maintain the position for a few minutes—the longer the better—while your mind is in a peaceful, pleasant, or meditative state."

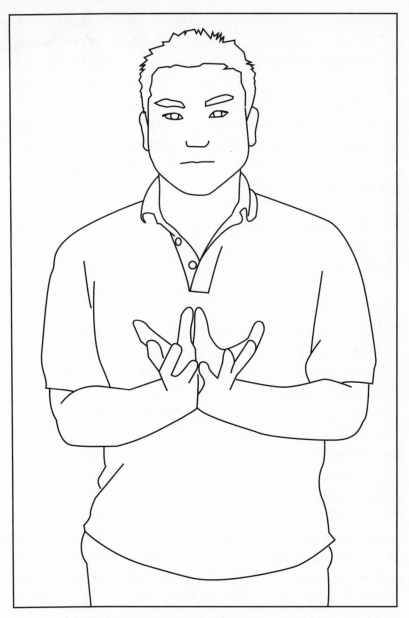

Figure 7.2 Xiu Lian body power technique

Meditation for Emotional Cleansing

While most people associate meditation with religion, this simple, powerful act transcends religious beliefs. Meditation is a brief vacation from the stresses of day-to-day life to centre your mind and create a feeling of peacefulness. The results are impressive.

In one study of forty-eight employees at a biotechnology company, half were trained in meditation and practised it for one hour a day, six days a week, using guided meditations that had been prerecorded on audiotapes. The other half of the participants did not meditate. Dr. Richard J. Davidson, of the University of Wisconsin, found that the meditators had greater electrical activity in their brains than the non-meditators. Some of the effects of meditation continued for up to four months after the participants stopped meditating.[6]

Other research shows improvements in mood, pain threshold, immune system activity, and bronchial and arterial smooth muscle tone, and a decrease in stress hormones and reversed effects of chronic stress.[7]

Daily practice offers the greatest benefits. Over time, it will become easier. By meditating on a regular basis you can train your mind to relax and release stress just by turning your attention to meditation.

There are several ways to meditate: breathing meditation, walking meditation, sitting meditation, mindfulness meditation, guided meditation, visualization, and prayer. Choose the type that has the most appeal and best fits with your lifestyle and health goals.

Breathing meditation is one of the easiest and most convenient forms of meditation. It can be done anywhere at almost any time, even if you only have several minutes. It requires no special equipment other than your lungs. You can do a breathing meditation while you are waiting in a doctor's office, grocery store lineup or at your desk. You can use a regular reminder throughout the day to help you remember to do deep breathing. For example, you could choose to take deep breaths at every red light while you are driving. You can take deep breaths on the hour throughout the day.

Focusing on your breath on a regular basis can help oxygenate your body and achieve a nearly immediate sense of relaxation.

Choose the form of meditation that most appeals to you and, as Nike would say, "Just do it." There are a million excuses for not meditating, starting with "I don't have time" or "I'm too tired" to "I don't know how to meditate." I believe that all these excuses and many others suggest unwillingness to make your health and life a priority. Principles 1 and 4 respectively suggest "You are the director of your life" and "Nurture and respect yourself."

Make time for meditation, even if it is on the bus ride home from work, or while you are sitting in your office, but do it daily. The rewards are far greater than the time and effort it takes to meditate. In fact, you will soon discover that meditation requires little or no effort at all.

Here is a simple meditation exercise:

You can play peaceful background music while performing this meditation or you can have silence, whichever you prefer.

1. Sit in a comfortable position where you will not be disturbed. If you have children, it is important to teach them to respect your quiet time. Taking time to recharge and release stress will allow you to be a better parent. Close your eyes. Keep your head upright and shoulders relaxed.
2. Begin by breathing deeply and steadily. Do not force your breathing. Simply breathe as deeply as you can comfortably. Observe your breath.
3. Begin to allow your breath to expand your abdomen. Comfortably expand your abdomen with each inhalation and then release the abdomen with every exhalation.
4. Continue breathing deeply for at least five minutes, the longer the better.

Practise this meditation daily, increasing the amount of time each day. You can also purchase excellent guided meditation CDs, cassettes, videos, and DVDs to help with your meditation practice.

Energy Medicine for Emotional Detoxification

You learned about energy and the importance of maintaining strong and balanced energies in Chapter 6. Dr. Candace Pert, in her book *Molecules of Emotion: The Science Behind Mind-Body Medicine*, explains that emotions can and do become stored in our bodies at the cellular level.

Donna Eden and David Feinstein in their book, *Energy Medicine*, explain stress this way: "When we are experiencing intense stress, we are not biologically programmed to sit around thinking about our problems. Your forebrain is not even well designed for saving you from immediate danger; your reptilian brain structure is far better organized for producing quick and effective defensive responses. But it doesn't distinguish whether the alarm was set off by a physical threat, a relationship spat, pressure on the job, or a myriad of daily irritations. When the crisis response is needlessly engaged, not only is it useless in helping you survive, it plays havoc with your health and tranquillity."

You can help your body to eliminate stresses that may be stored within by performing this simple exercise, which Eden and Feinstein describe in their book:

Holding a stressful memory in your mind while touching specific spots on your head, called neurovascular holding points, conditions primitive brain centers to have a composed rather than an emergency response to the memory. By resetting your nervous system in this way, the stress response cycle is not activated when the memory occurs.

1. Lightly place your fingertips on your forehead, covering the frontal eminences (the bumps on your forehead directly above your eyes);

2. Put your thumbs on your temples next to your eyes, breathing deeply;
3. As the blood returns to your forebrain over the next few minutes, you will find yourself beginning to think more clearly. It is that simple![8]

Holding these points for three to five minutes while fully thinking about and feeling the negative stressor helps affect blood circulation to the forebrain and throughout the body.

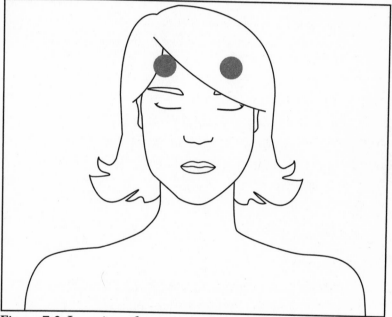

Figure 7.3 Location of neurovascular holding points

Bach Flower Therapy for Emotional Cleansing

Dr. Edward Bach, a British medical doctor and bacteriologist, discovered a system of treating emotional imbalances using the "essence" of flowers. He had observed that many of his patients' emotional difficulties seemed to be having a negative effect on their physical health.

In search of a way to help them and after many years of studying wild flowers in England, he developed remedies to work on mental and emotional fixations.

The basic principle of this form of therapy is simple: people with fearful, worried, or depressed mental states heal more slowly and less completely than do those with positive, cheerful, and hopeful states of mind.

To incorporate Bach flower remedies into your detox program, go through the list below and the description of personality characteristics to find the one or two remedies whose descriptions most resemble your feelings or personality at this stage in your life. You may notice descriptions that sound like your personality years ago; however, unless that description also fits you at this stage of your life, you need not use it. We are working on emotions you are currently experiencing.

The remedies, which are in the form of liquids, usually come in small dropper bottles. Follow the directions on the bottle or place several drops under your tongue or in a glass of water and sip throughout the day.

Agrimony—suffers a lot internally, but keeps it hidden
Aspen—fear of unknown things
Beech—arrogant, critical, and intolerant
Centaury—weak-willed, subservient, and easily used
Cerato—lack of self-confidence, asks advice
Cherry plum—fear of going crazy, losing control, or causing harm, violent temper
Chestnut bud—fails to learn by experience, repeats mistakes
Chicory—overpossessive, selfish, and attention-seeking
Clematis—absentminded, dreamy, and mentally escapist
Crab apple—self-dislike, feels unclean

Elm—temporary inadequacy

Gentian—depression with known cause, easily discouraged

Gorse—depression, all seems pointless

Heather—obsessed with own problems

Holly—jealousy, suspicion, revenge, hate

Honeysuckle—living in the past

Hornbeam—procrastinators

Impatiens—impatient

Larch—depression, inferiority, expects to fail

Mimulus—fear of known things

Mustard—deep depression without reason

Oak—brave, plodders, determined

Olive—mental and physical exhaustion

Pine—guilt, self-blame

Red chestnut—fear for others

Rescue Remedy—a combination of cherry plum, clematis, impatiens, and Star of Bethlehem used for shock, trauma, and external and internal first aid

Rock rose—terror, panic

Rock water—self-demanding, self-denial

Scleranthus—indecision, mood swings

Star of Bethlehem—shock

Sweet chestnut—despair, no hope left

Vervain—fanatical, tense, overenthusiastic

Vine—ambitious, tyrannical, demanding, unbending, power-seeking

Walnut—the "link" breaker, for times of change

Water violet—reserve, pride, reliability

White chestnut—persistent thoughts and mental chatter

Wild oat—helps define goals

Wild rose—apathetic slackers, unambitious; and

Willow—bitter, resentful.[9]

Although it is not necessary to do all the suggested exercises and practices provided in this chapter, a combination of any of journalling, qigong breathing exercises, holding the neurovascular points on your forehead, meditating, and using Bach flower remedies can provide emotional cleansing to alleviate pent-up emotions or old wounds that may be stored in your cellular memory, or to simply feel more capable of handling stress.

In this chapter you learned
+ The 10 Emotional Detox Principles
+ A simple meditation/breathing exercise that you can use any time
+ Ancient Chinese qigong exercises
+ The benefits of meditating and incorporating energy exercises into your life
+ The effects of toxic people in our lives and suggestions for dealing with them

References

1. Michael Murray, "Good Health and Optimism Go Hand in Hand," *Health & Wellness Newsletter*, Spring 2004.

2. Murray, "Good Health and Optimism Go Hand in Hand."

3. Murray, "Good Health and Optimism Go Hand in Hand."

4. Richard Gerber, *Vibrational Medicine for the 21st Century: The Complete Guide to Energy Healing and Spiritual Transformation* (New York, NY: Eagle Brook, 2000).

5. Zhi Gang Sha, *Power Healing* (San Francisco, CA: HarperCollins Publishers, Inc., 2002).

6. "Brain Scans, Blood Tests Show Positive Effects of Meditation," *Health Behavior News Service*, August 16, 2003.

7. Tin Htut, "The Effects of Meditation on the Body," *Triplegem.plus.com*. September 18, 1999.

8. Donna Eden and David Feinstein, *Energy Medicine* (New York, NY: Jeremy P. Tarcher/Penguin Books, 1998).

9. Lisha Simester, *The Natural Health Bible* (North Vancouver: Whitecap Books, 2001).

CHAPTER 8

Targeting the Kidneys and Intestines

"Of one thing I am certain, the body is not the measure of healing—peace is the measure."

George Melton

In this chapter you will learn
- How the kidneys, urinary tract, and intestines contribute to good health
- The signs that the kidneys, urinary tract, and intestines need cleansing
- How to cleanse the kidneys, urinary tract and intestines using food, herbs, and energy medicine

In Chapter 5 you learned many of the essentials for detoxifying your body to start experiencing greater energy, mental clarity, and other health improvements. Now I am going to explain how you can reap even greater rewards by finding your body's weakest detoxification systems so you can target your efforts there.

As you learned earlier, you can stay at any of the four phases for longer than the prescribed week, to help cleanse, strengthen, and tone these systems. In addition, you can further strengthen these systems by targeting them after you finish *The 4-Week Ultimate Body Detox Plan*. You can also incorporate some of the nutritional, herbal, and other types of therapies in the next five chapters into the 4-Week Plan. Let's examine the various organs and organ systems in each phase so you have a better understanding of their functioning, then we'll learn how to further target your efforts to maximize your results.

The four phases of *The 4-Week Ultimate Body Detox Plan* are these:

Phase 1: Cleansing the Kidneys and Bowels

Phase 2: Cleansing the Lymphatic System (and Cellulite)

Phase 3: Cleansing the Liver and Gallbladder (and Fat Deposits

Phase 4: Cleansing the Blood, Lungs, and Skin

I will provide nutritional advice, herbal suggestions, and ideas for other natural means to help your body most effectively cleanse and heal.

I have spoken to many salespeople regarding herbs, and many will tell you that everything you need for your treatment is found in whatever herb they are trying to push that month. That is simply not true. Some herbs are better than others for a specific purpose. There is no single herb that does everything. One herb may be adequate for the needs of a particular person but not for everyone. To help you determine whether you require additional cleansing of a particular organ system, I have included quizzes you can take. This is an area where *The 4-Week Ultimate Body Detox Plan* can be customized to suit you and your individual needs.

If you are pregnant or have a serious health condition, consult a medical doctor before using any herbs. Consult a herbalist before combining two or more herbs or while taking medication with herbs. Avoid long-term use of any herb (longer than three weeks) without first consulting a qualified herbalist.

YOUR KIDNEYS AND URINARY TRACT

During Phase 1 we targeted the kidneys, urinary system, and the small and large intestines. As you learned earlier, your kidneys are two small organs in the abdominal area that have several main functions: they strive to maintain balance in your body, particularly fluid and sodium balances; excrete toxins in urine; and regulate blood pressure through hormone production. Cleansing the kidneys also has the additional effect of better enabling them to regulate blood pressure because the kidneys secrete a hormone to fulfil that function.

The kidneys allow many substances to enter the urine, where they can be filtered and reabsorbed if they are items your body needs, such as minerals.

Many toxins are created within your body merely as by-products of normal metabolic functions. These are excreted in the urine, via the kidneys, provided the kidneys can adequately filter these substances.

Since kidneys are heavily involved with regulating your body's mineral and water balance, and thereby help to prevent your cells from becoming dehydrated or overhydrated, it is critical to help them perform optimally.

During this program, we started by cleansing the kidneys. The health of all the other organs in the body is dependent on the kidneys functioning well. If they are functioning up to par, they are able to remove toxins before most of the other detox organs need to start their work. If the kidneys are unable to remove toxins from the blood, toxins are deposited in your tissues. Pain and inflammation or weight gain may be the result.

The kidneys are responsible for eliminating waste products when high-protein foods are broken down into their key components, called amino acids. The waste products of metabolizing these products include urea and ammonia. These substances can become toxic if the kidneys cannot handle the amount of protein in the diet. This is an important issue. High animal-protein diets are currently a massive fad. Although these popular diets may encourage quick and seemingly effortless weight loss, it comes at a price—overburdened kidneys. I conduct urine tests in my laboratory and can almost always tell when a person is following a high animal-protein diet because the urine shows signs of toxicity and kidney stress. Short-term gain should not cause long-term pain. Weight loss should not come at the potential cost of disease. A far superior approach to weight loss is to try to eat well. Throughout this book, you will learn many easy-to-maintain ways to improve your eating habits.

Kidney and Urinary Tract Stress Quiz

Are you suffering from any of the following problems?

Back pain

Blood in your urine

Cloudy urine

Congestive heart failure

Dark-coloured urine

Difficult, frequent, or painful urination

Edema or bloating

Frequent chills, fevers, or nausea

High blood pressure

Kidney or bladder cancer

Kidney stones

Puffiness around the eyes

Swollen fingers, ankles, legs, etc.

If you answered yes to any of these questions, your kidneys and urinary tract could use further detoxification.

Eat for Clean Kidneys and Urinary Tract

Since the kidneys work to balance the acidity and alkalinity in your body, it is imperative to lighten the acid load by improving your diet. You will want to eat a diet rich in alkaline foods such as fresh raw fruits and raw or cooked vegetables. Cooked fruit becomes acidic and should be avoided while cleansing the urinary tract.

All the kidney's jobs require enough water. The most common type of stress that the kidneys face is dehydration due to lack of water intake. If you do not drink enough water, your kidneys will not be able to perform their many important functions, and your cells will become dehydrated, making virtually every function in your body less efficient. It is important to drink enough water to adequately bathe your cells in fluid to enable them to function properly. A simple way to improve kidney function is to drink large amounts of water: at least two litres per day, and more to assist with cleansing.

Kidney health depends on many factors but can be affected by diet, exercise, stress, cardiovascular disease, genetic weaknesses, infections, and kidney stones.

One of the best ways to assist your kidneys and urinary tract to improve their functioning is to reduce your intake of salt and increase your consumption of potassium-rich foods. A diet that is rich in nutrients, including potassium, but other minerals as well, is beneficial to the kidneys. Unfortunately, much of our produce supply is quickly losing minerals due to substandard soil and today's agricultural practices. Research consistently proves that organic fruits and vegetables contain substantially greater quantities of vitamins and minerals than their conventional counterparts. Opt for organic produce wherever possible.

Cranberries and cranberry juice are powerful cleansers of the kidneys and urinary tract. Cranberries contain a substance called arbutin, which pulls excess fluid from your tissues to be eliminated through your kidneys.[1] In addition, cranberries and their juice help break down the fatty deposits in the lymphatic system that lead to cellulite. It improves the cleansing ability of the body's tissues. I have included cranberry juice in this chapter, but you will find that it is continued through Phase 2 of the program, "Targeting Your Lymphatic System and Cellulite" as well.

Herbs for Deep Cleansing Your Kidneys and Urinary Tract

Herbs that increase the flow of urine are beneficial to the kidneys and urinary tract. Some of the best herbs for this purpose include dandelion, cleavers, boldo, buchu, couchgrass, bearberry, birch, celery seed, juniper, and one of my favourites, yarrow.

Dandelion (*Taraxacum officinale*)

Dandelion has a bad reputation as nothing more than a pesky weed. Like most other weeds that people regard as a mere nuisance, it has scientifically proven medicinal properties. We spend billions, if not trillions, of dollars searching for the one little miracle pill that will cure what ails us, while Mother Nature has provided medicine right beneath our noses. If we'd only stop whining about the "weeds" we have to deal with and start cultivating these powerful healing herbs, we'd be much healthier. I am not suggesting that you start eating dandelions off your lawn, although it is something that is possible with a little knowledge and the assurance of an organic lawn.

An Arabian doctor first recorded dandelion's curative properties in the tenth century. Dandelion was once called "piddley bed" because of its ability to increase urine flow. The French have a less tactful name for the plant as well. It is called "pissenlit." For those of you who don't speak any French, I'll let you know that "en lit" means "in bed." I'll leave you to figure out the rest.

Dandelion is one of the best detoxification and healing herbs. The leaves tend to be best for cleansing the kidneys, but the root can be used as well. You will learn more about dandelion root below, since it is beneficial for the liver. Unlike pharmaceutical diuretics that can cause mineral depletion and, ultimately, dehydration, dandelion comes with a high supply of potassium and calcium to help prevent this problem. Dandelion is also packed with protein, healthy sugars, vitamins A and C, iron, and other minerals, vitamins, and nutrients. Use one teaspoon of the dried leaves per cup of water to make an infusion. Drink one cup, three times daily. If you have gallstones or obstructed bile ducts, consult a holistic physician before using dandelion.

Cleavers (*also known as Goosegrass or Grip Grass*)
Don't be alarmed by the name of this herb—it is actually an amazing herb for the kidneys. It helps the kidneys eliminate toxins and waste fluids, thereby draining excess toxins and fluid from the tissues. For cleavers tea, use two to three teaspoons of the dried herb per cup of water. Drink one cup three times daily. Alternatively use a half to one teaspoon of tincture three times per day. Avoid using cleavers if you suffer from diabetes or have diabetic tendencies.

Boldo (*Peumus boldo*)
This unusual-sounding herb helps deal with excess fluid in the tissues by strengthening the kidney's ability to eliminate toxins. Boldo also helps with urinary tract infections such as cystitis. If you are prone to these types of infections, or are uncertain whether an older infection ever healed fully, then boldo is one of the herbs of choice. While cleansing the urinary tract, it also helps to soothe mucous membranes that line the bladder and urethra. Make an infusion from one teaspoon of dried leaves to one cup of boiling water. Let sit for five to ten minutes. Drink one cup, three times per day. Alternatively, take 1/4 teaspoon of the tincture three times daily.

Buchu (*Agathosma betulina*)

Buchu is a fabulous herb for the kidneys. It helps increase urinary flow, thereby helping the kidneys to eliminate toxins. It also helps with urinary tract infections. Its main use is for the kidneys and urinary tract, unlike many other herbs that also tend to work on different parts of the body. As a result, it is beneficial for conditions such as cystitis, urethritis, prostatitis, and burning and painful urination. Use one teaspoon of dried leaves per cup of water. Drink one cup three times daily.

Couchgrass (*Agropyron repens*)

This is not the grass that grows beneath the feet of couch potatoes. This cleansing and healing herb is also helpful for many inflammatory conditions of the urinary tract, including cystitis, urethritis, prostatitis, prostate hypertrophy, and kidney stones and gravel. Like dandelion, it is rich in potassium. Allow two teaspoons of dried herb per cup of water. Bring to a boil. Reduce the heat and allow to simmer for twenty minutes. Strain. Drink one cup three times per day. Alternatively, take 1 to 1-1/2 teaspoons of tincture twice daily.

Bearberry (*Arctostaphylos Uva ursi*)

Bearberry helps primarily with infections and kidney stones or gravel, but it is also helpful with vaginal infections and vaginitis. It is an excellent kidney and urinary tract cleanser, particularly if there is inflammation in these areas. Consult an herbalist before using this herb in combination with others. Avoid large doses, which can lead to nausea or vomiting. For an infusion, use one teaspoon of the dried leaves per cup of boiling water. Allow the mixture to sit for twenty minutes. Drink one cup, three times daily.

Birch (*Betula pendula, also known as Silver Birch*)

In addition to helping with urinary tract infections, birch leaves and bark are good for reducing fluid retention in the body, and for rheumatism and arthritis. It helps to remove excess fluid from the body's tissues and eases pain. For an infusion, use one to two teaspoons of the dried leaves per cup of boiling water. Allow the mixture to sit for twenty minutes. Drink one cup, three times daily. Alternatively, take 1/4 to 1/2 teaspoon of the tincture three times per day.

Celery Seed (*Apium graveolens*)

Not only do celery seeds provide excellent assistance with urinary tract cleansing and infections, but James Duke, author of *The Green Pharmacy*, found more than twenty anti-inflammatory compounds in celery and celery seeds, including a substance called apigenin, which is powerful in its anti-inflammatory action. Incidentally, Hildegard von Bingen, a writer, scientist, musician, nun, and visionary, wrote about celery's anti-inflammatory properties over nine hundred years ago.

In addition to taking celery seeds as a herbal supplement or in herb teas, you can also cook with them. Simply add them to soups and stews or use them as a salt substitute in many recipes. One of my favourite appetizers is celery bread. See Chapter 13: The Ultimate Body Detox Plan Recipes.

Celery seeds have a slightly salty taste like celery but don't let their good taste fool you. They are potent medicine. They help with arthritis, rheumatism, and gout while cleansing the kidneys and helping to alleviate infections. Use one to two teaspoons of freshly crushed celery seeds per cup of boiling water to make a tea that not only helps with cleansing the urinary tract but also helps normalize high blood pressure and blood sugar levels, ease the pain of gout and arthritis, and alleviate bloating during menstruation.

Avoid eating or taking celery seeds while pregnant.

Juniper (*Juniperus, various species*)

Juniper berries are mildly cleansing and restorative of the kidneys. The other herbs mentioned above are certainly more powerful, but juniper is also effective for arthritis and rheumatism as well as generalized muscular and joint pain. Be sure to work with an herbalist if you choose to use this herb because the berries can be toxic in large amounts. Avoid using juniper berries if you are pregnant or have any inflammatory disorder of the kidneys. Use one teaspoon of dried juniper berries per cup of boiling water. Allow to infuse for at least ten minutes. Drink one cup, three times daily. Alternatively, take one teaspoon of tincture, three times daily or take as directed on the package.

Yarrow (*Achillea millefolium*)

The leaves, stems, and flowers of this plant make an effective remedy for cleansing the kidneys, while promoting cleansing of the skin through perspiration, helping to regulate high blood pressure, and improving immune system function. I always go wildcrafting (to collect herbs in the wilderness or other areas they are found) to collect wild yarrow during the summer months to dry and store for use throughout the year. Use one teaspoon of the dried herb per cup of boiling water. Drink one cup three times per day.

Energy Exercises to Supercharge Your Kidney Cleansing

As you learned in Chapter 6, there are points along energy pathways called acupressure points that can be used for healing the body. To supercharge your kidney cleansing efforts, Donna Eden and David Feinstein, the authors of *Energy Medicine*, recommend the following acupressure points. Use the points for the kidneys and the bladder to help detoxify the whole urinary tract.

Apply firm pressure to the following points. Hold each point for a minute or two. You can work on both sides simultaneously. For example, Kidney 1 is located in a slight depression beneath the balls of both feet, described below. You can apply pressure to this point on both feet at the same time. There are two sets of points for each organ. The exercise is most effective if you apply pressure to the points in the order I give them below.

If you are pregnant, avoid using the point Stomach 36 and consult an acupuncturist before proceeding with acupressure.

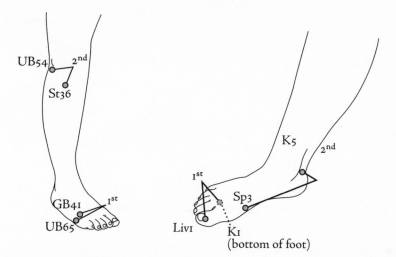

Figure 8.1 Kidney acupressure points & urinary bladder acupressure points

For the kidneys, use the following points:

+ Liver 1 (Liv 1) is located on the edge of the big toe near the bottom corner of the toenail, on the edge near the second toe.
+ Kidney 1 (K 1) is located on the base of the ball of the foot. This point is found in a slight depression.

Then:

+ Spleen 3 (Sp 3) is located on the inside of the foot, at the base of the protrusion behind the big toe.
+ Kidney 5 (K 5) is located just behind the ankle bone, on the inside of the foot.

For the bladder, use the following points:

- Gallbladder 41 (GB 41) is located on the top of the foot toward the outside edge, about an inch and a half above the fourth toe (the toe nearest the little toe).
- Urinary Bladder 65 (UB 65) is located on the outside edge of the foot, about an inch below the base of the little toe.

Then:

- Stomach 36 (St 36) is located in the space where the two lower leg bones meet just below and to the outer edge of the kneecap.
- Urinary Bladder 54 (UB 54) is located toward the outside edge of the base of the knee.

YOUR INTESTINAL TRACT

You are what you eat, according to the old adage. But, I think "you are what you digest, assimilate, and absorb" is an important addition to the saying. After all, what you eat, digest, assimilate, and absorb will become the building blocks of every cell in your body.

Digestion 101[2]

I discussed digestion earlier, but it's important to review it here. Digestion begins in the mouth. The act of chewing stimulates the digestive juices, both in the mouth as well as lower in the digestive tract. The saliva in the mouth contains an enzyme called amylase that starts the digestion of starchy foods such as pasta, rice, potatoes, and bread. Your mother may have told you to "chew your food well"—she was right. Foods need time to mingle with this enzyme to be properly broken down. If you gulp your food down quickly, you are missing a vital stage of the digestion process.

Once you swallow, the food travels down a tube called the esophagus to the stomach. The stomach secretes a powerful acid that starts the digestion of protein-based foods such as meat, fish, legumes, dairy products, nuts, and seeds. This acid is so powerful that it would burn a hole through your skin if it were located anywhere but the stomach. The stomach contains a thick coat of mucus that acts as a barrier.

After food leaves the stomach, it passes into the small intestine. The intestinal tract is one of the most important detox systems in the body. The approximately twenty-two-foot-long small intestine aids with food digestion. It also allows nutrients and water to be absorbed into the bloodstream. The small intestine also produces some digestive enzymes: peptidase breaks down protein, maltase breaks down maltose (a form of sugar), and sucrase breaks down sucrose (another form of sugar). Some people's intestines also secrete lactase to break down lactose (milk sugar). The pancreas secretes many enzymes into the small intestine to aid in the digestive process. The gall bladder secretes bile—a digestive juice produced by the liver—into the small intestines to assist with fat digestion. Nutrients are absorbed into the bloodstream through the lining of the small intestine.

Then the remaining food is passed down to the large intestine. At this point, the waste matter is mostly liquid. The large intestine, which is about five feet long and two and a half inches across, does not digest food. Instead it absorbs substances such as vitamins B1, B2, B12, and K, produced by healthy bacteria found in undigested waste matter. The large intestine also helps maintain the body's fluid balance by absorbing about 90 percent of the water in undigested waste.

The food molecules that are absorbed into the blood through the intestinal walls are transferred to the liver by the bloodstream. There, some food molecules are broken down further while others are converted into fuel that can be stored by the body.

Toxins move from the blood into the intestines, where they are detoxified, eliminated, or reabsorbed into the bloodstream. Toxins are also sent to the liver for detoxification. The remaining waste product of the food, which can contain some toxins, is then eliminated.

The average person's low-fibre, low-water, high-protein, high-sugar, and high-fat diet disrupts the natural processes in the intestines. Lack of fibre in the diet results in inadequate bulk to push digested food through the intestines. Low water also delays the process and disrupts the natural fluid balance in the body. High amounts of protein create acidity in the intestines that allow harmful bacteria to overgrow. Excess sugar can cause harmful bacteria or fungi to overgrow in the intestines, preventing healthy bacteria from producing the nutrients the body needs. When harmful bacteria or fungi overgrow, health can be negatively affected.

Inefficient elimination allows toxins to back up and be absorbed through the walls of the intestines into the blood, where they can cause problems. Toxin reabsorption can also occur when you avoid Nature's call. When you feel like you have to use the bathroom, go immediately. Do not wait. Many experts believe that holding back the urge to have a bowel movement is linked with cellulite, in addition to many dangerous toxins being absorbed into your bloodstream.

Many studies show the link between intestinal toxicity and health problems. The medical journal *The Lancet* reported a study that showed the link between poor intestinal health and breast disease. Out of 1,500 women, the study found less breast disease in those who had daily bowel movements. The women who had two or fewer bowel movements per week had four times the likelihood of breast disease.[3]

Another study reported in the *American Journal of Public Health* of over 7,000 women found an increased incidence of breast cancer in women who experienced constipation, infrequent bowel movements, or hard stools.[4]

Ancient Egyptians also understood the importance of intestinal health on overall health. They had seven levels of doctors. The highest level was the doctor who was reserved for royalty in Egypt. Only a physician who specialized in intestinal health could hold the position of top doctor. The title for the prestigious position translates as "The Guardian of the Royal Ass."[5]

Intestinal Stress Quiz

Do you suffer from any of the following?[26]

Acne

Allergies

Anxiety

Appendicitis

Autoimmune disorders

Back pain

Bladder or vaginal infections

Brain fog (lack of mental clarity)

Breast cancer

Breast tenderness

Brittle nails or hair

Cancer

Candida albicans overgrowth

Chronic fatigue syndrome

Coated tongue

Colon cancer

Constipation

Crohn's disease

Depression

Diarrhea

Diverticulosis

Earaches

Eczema or psoriasis

Fatigue

Fibromyalgia

Flatulence

Food sensitivities

Frequent sore throats

Headaches or migraines

High cholesterol

Infections

Insomnia

Intestinal polyps

Irritability

Irritable bowel syndrome

Mood swings

Muscle or joint pain

Nausea and bloating

Premenstrual syndrome

Protruding abdomen

Recurrent fevers

Sinus problems

Skin problems

Unpleasant breath or body odour

Vaginitis

Eat for a Clean Intestinal Tract[7]

Before we delve into the factors that help ensure a clean intestinal tract, let's look at some of the causes of poor digestion. Once we have a better idea about the factors that contribute to poor digestion, we can work to improve digestion. Once digestion is improved, we have eliminated half the battle for a clean intestinal tract.

Failure to chew food properly is a major contributor to poor digestion and a backed-up intestinal system. This is usually the result of eating too quickly or on the run. Because the rest of the digestive system depends on food being properly chewed, inadequate chewing may result in indigestion or other uncomfortable symptoms later. So the first step to a cleaner intestinal tract is to chew your food well.

Drinking large amounts of fluids with meals (drinking too much at mealtimes) dilutes the digestive secretions and enzymes, thereby reducing their efficiency. In addition, a mechanism in the stomach tells it when to move food onward in the digestive tract. When food has been adequately broken down by the acid medium in the stomach, the stomach becomes slightly less acidic. This is a signal the body uses to inform the stomach that its job is done. Drinking with meals can improperly trick the stomach into thinking it has finished digestion because the fluids dilute the acid. This makes the stomach dump the food prematurely into the small intestines. The small intestines cannot perform the work of the stomach. Only the stomach can do the stomach's work, so avoid drinking at mealtimes. If you have supplements to take with food, drink only enough to help swallow them. It is better to drink one-half hour before or one to two hours after meals.

Conversely, not drinking enough water between meals can result in inadequate water in the intestines, which means hard stools that are difficult to pass and a slow transit time in the intestines. Toxins can get backed up and be reabsorbed into the bloodstream. Caffeinated beverages dehydrate the body so it is imperative to drink an additional two cups of water for every cup of a caffeinated beverage. Drink plenty of pure water between meals.

The digestive system was not designed for many of the heavy and complex meals we eat. The larger the meal, the less likely the body can digest it properly. Also, having complex meals made up of many different ingredients can be too difficult for the body's enzymes to adequately handle. Consider what you may have learned in high school chemistry. Because proteins require an acid medium and carbohydrates (starches) require an alkaline medium for digestion, mixing the two can neutralize the digestive juices required for each. The result: inadequate digestion. Eat small meals and occasional snacks to avoid overloading the digestive tract.

Emotional or mental stress impairs the function of the digestive system. That is why it is best not to eat when you are upset. Avoid eating while you are very stressed.

Because digestive processes slow down in the later part of the day, eating late can mean that the body does not adequately digest meals.

Some of the main problems with eating late include weight gain, gas, heartburn, indigestion, and bloating. Avoid eating for two to three hours before bedtime and avoid heavy meals late in the day.

As we age, we tend to produce fewer digestive enzymes and less hydrochloric acid in the stomach. This inadequacy results in improper digestion or digestive problems, along with other health concerns such as allergies, flatulence, weight gain, and nutrient deficiencies. At least half of your meal should be raw. This is quite easy to accomplish when you eat a large raw salad with both lunch and dinner.

Eating foods devoid of enzymes (all cooked foods, canned foods, fried foods, packaged foods, fast foods, basically, anything that is not raw) can cause incomplete digestion and depletion of your body's own internal digestive enzymes. Incomplete digestion can cause foods to decay, promoting the growth of harmful bacteria, fungi, and parasites. In addition to eating a high amount of raw foods, you can also take a digestive enzyme with every meal, particularly with any meals that contain cooked food.

Include foods that contain essential fatty acids in your daily diet. These foods, such as cold-pressed flax oil and extra-virgin olive oil, help lubricate your intestinal tract.

Eating refined, processed, fried, salted, or packaged foods can cause constipation. Foods that are made with white sugar, white flour, excess salt, unhealthy fats, and synthetic chemicals are basically "empty foods" that cause you to feel full without providing the fibre, water, vitamins, minerals, enzymes, and other nutrients your body needs. The result is constipation and malnourishment. Avoid these empty foods while you are doing an intestinal cleanse.

Eating excessive animal products, all of which are devoid of fibre, can also make you feel full without providing adequate fibre. These animal products include beef, poultry, fish, seafood, dairy products, and others. During your cleanse, refrain from eating meat, dairy, and all animal products.

I have mentioned constipation and how it contributes to disease. But what exactly constitutes constipation? Ideally, you should have two to three large bowel movements *per day*. I am sure many people will balk at the idea of having this many bowel movements. We live in a chronically constipated society, based on unhealthy eating habits. Bear with me while I delve further into a topic that is uncomfortable for many people. It is important to understand this topic better since it is so critical to good health. Your stools should be well-formed, large, and slightly soft. Hard, small, or misshapen bowel movements suggest that you need to put more effort into cleansing the intestines, as well as eating a high-fibre, high-nutrient, and high-water diet.

Harmful bacteria overgrowth in the intestines impedes the healthy flora that are needed there to ensure you properly absorb the nutrients in your food. As many as four hundred different strains of bacteria can inhabit the intestines. There can be 100 trillion microorganisms living in your intestines. Ideally, the ratio should be approximately 85 percent good bacteria to 15 percent pathogenic bacteria.[8] For many people, the ratio is the opposite. This incorrect balance between good and pathogenic bacteria is referred to as dysbiosis. Eating a diet high in sugar and animal protein is one reason for the imbalance. Taking antibiotics for various health concerns also causes the harmful pathogens to become stronger and more resistant, and they become harder to eliminate. It is important to deal with any problems with bacterial or fungal overgrowth.

At least 150 species of yeasts are known as candida, but one particular one that frequently tends to become overgrown in the intestines is *Candida albicans*. The condition is referred to as candidiasis. Candida releases over eighty known toxins. These toxins weaken the defences of the body and can cause the mucous membranes of the gut to leak, allowing undigested protein molecules to be absorbed into the bloodstream. This, in turn, can result in allergic reactions and food and chemical sensitivities.

Taking a nutritional supplement of beneficial bacteria known as probiotics is helpful for cleansing the intestines and dealing with candida. Regardless of whether you suspect candida overgrowth, you would likely benefit from a probiotic supplement. The main strains of beneficial bacteria include *Lactobacillus acidophilus*, *Bifidobacterium bifidum*, *Lactobacillus bulgaricus*, *Lactobacillus sporogenes*, *Lactobacillus salivarius*, and *Lactobacillus plantarum*. You will sometimes see "lactobacillus" listed on the label of a nutritional supplement as "L." For example, "L. bifidum."

Many factors lead to candida overgrowth, including the following:[9]

Alcohol intake (wine, beer, champagne, etc.)
Antibiotics
Birth control pills
Blood sugar imbalances
Consumption of foods that contain antibiotics and hormones
    (meat, chicken, dairy products)
Excessive sugar intake
High bread, wheat, or yeast consumption
Immunosuppressive drugs
    (steroids, cortisone, etc.)
Mercury amalgam dental fillings
Multiple sexual partners
Nutritional deficiencies
Poor diet
Recreational drug use
Stress
Toxic exposures, especially to mold
Weakened immunity

Studies in rats found that candida stimulates histamine production.[10] Histamine is a substance in the body that is released typically in response to an allergen. This research indicates that candida over-growth may be an underlying factor in some allergic reactions. Some experts estimate that 80 percent of people with multiple allergies have candida overgrowth.

Candida also produces hormone-like substances that interfere with normal hormone production.[11] These hormone-like substances can disrupt the body's normal hormone balance, particularly in women.

A diet deficient in essential nutrients such as vitamins, amino acids, and essential fatty acids weakens the immune system and can lead to candida overgrowth.

Although the intestines are the primary site for candida over-growth, candida can spread throughout the body. Cleansing the intestines and following a nutritional program that starves candida is the best way to deal with this insidious pathogen. To help you determine whether candida may be a problem for you, take the following Candida Quiz.

Candida Quiz

There are many symptoms of yeast overgrowth. Do you suffer from any of the following?[12]

Acne, psoriasis, eczema, rashes, or hives

Allergies

Anal, vaginal or jock itch

Anemia

Anxiety

Asthma

Athlete's foot

Attention Deficit Disorder (ADD) or Attention Deficit and Hyperactivity Disorder (ADHD)

Autism

Bloating and flatulence

Body odour or bad breath
Brain fog or memory lapses
Chemical sensitivities
Constipation or diarrhea
Cravings for sweets, bread, or alcohol
Crohn's disease
Depression
Difficulty gaining or losing weight
Diminished libido
Fatigue that sleep doesn't help
Fibromyalgia
Food sensitivities
Headaches, especially frequent
Heartburn
Hormonal imbalances
Hypoglycemia
Immune dysfunction
Indecisiveness
Insomnia
Irritable bowel syndrome
Joint or muscle aches
Lack of concentration
Mood swings or irritability
Nasal congestion
Premenstrual syndrome
Recurrent bladder, sinus, vaginal yeast, or respiratory infections
Thyroid conditions
Unexplained weight changes

If you answered yes to any of these questions, you may be suffering from candida overgrowth and might benefit from the intestinal cleansing suggestions above as well as the candida cleansing suggestions below.

Candida Cleansing

If you are trying to rebalance your intestinal flora to eliminate a candida overgrowth, follow the numerous dietary and nutritional suggestions above, as well as the following ones.

Refrain from eating sugar, foods with yeast, and alcohol. That includes all sweets, breads made with yeast, and alcoholic beverages, especially wine and beer. Also, avoid dairy products (especially cheeses). Refrain from eating foods that typically have molds or yeasts present on them, including peanuts and all types of vinegar except apple cider vinegar. Apple cider vinegar actually helps kill candida bacteria.

Eat plenty of fruits and vegetables, both steamed and raw.

Eat some high-protein foods at each meal. That includes beans and legumes, soy milk, organic eggs, and tofu.

Eat foods such as garlic, onions, scallions, and horseradish, all of which destroy harmful yeasts and parasites. Season your food with herbs that have similar effects, including basil, dill, oregano, and ginger.

Choose anti-parasitic herbs from those mentioned below to help reduce candida overgrowth in the intestines.

Clean Up Your Intestines

It is virtually impossible to have a well-functioning intestinal tract without doing exercise. Movement is critical to help the intestines keep digested food moving through your body. Exercise also keeps the abdominal muscles healthy and toned. Walking, yoga, rebounding, hiking, climbing stairs, dancing, gardening, and many other forms of exercise help keep you regular and your intestines cleansed. Exercise for at least thirty minutes a day, five days a week.

Magnesium (the mineral) is one of nature's best natural and gentle laxatives. It adds water to the stool to assist with its easy elimination from the body.[13] Eat foods that are high in magnesium, such as apples, figs, peaches, kale, chard, celery, beet greens, brown rice, sesame seeds, sunflower seeds, almonds, and soybeans. In addition, take 400 milligrams of magnesium per day to supplement your diet.

Herbs for Deep Cleansing Your Intestinal Tract

Many herbs promote intestinal cleansing and the elimination of toxins and built-up fecal matter; however, not all herbs are suitable for taking for long periods of time. Some people take herbs such as senna and cascara sagrada, which are incredibly powerful and may be beneficial for acute problems but they are too aggressive for cleansing the bowels over the long term or for people whose bodies are more sensitive. I have selected herbs that are also powerful, but lack the harsh action of senna and cascara sagrada. The following ones are assertive without being aggressive.

Aloe Vera

Aloe vera juice acts as a natural stimulant to the colon.[14] Aloe vera has been used for over four thousand years for its ability to heal digestive tract ailments such as ulcers, dysentery, and kidney infections. It is full of amino acids, enzymes, chlorophyll, essential oils, vitamins and minerals, and other nutrients that are beneficial.

Aloe vera is known among herbalists as having antibacterial, antiviral, pain-killing, anti-inflammatory, fever-reducing, and cleansing properties. It also helps dilate capillaries and enhances normal cell growth, making it helpful for diseases such as arteriosclerosis and cancer.

Drink a quarter cup of aloe vera juice, twice a day. Note that aloe vera juice is not the same as the gel, which tends to be more concentrated. Avoid using "aloes" or "aloe latex" since its strong purgative action can be too harsh on the intestinal tract and result in severe cramping or diarrhea. Avoid taking aloe vera juice during pregnancy and lactation.

Slippery Elm Bark (*Ulmus rubra*)

Slippery elm bark soothes the lining of the intestines and helps minimize gas and bloating. For centuries it has been used as an expectorant and emollient. It is also high in mucilage,[15] thereby offering a protective coating to the digestive tract to help heal inflamed mucous membranes. It is helpful for disorders such as ulcers, gastritis, peptic ulcers, enteritis, colitis, diarrhea, and food poisoning. Make a decoction of slippery elm bark using two teaspoons of dried herb per cup of water. Drink one cup, three times daily. Alternatively, take one teaspoon of the tincture, three times daily. If you are prone to allergies, be cautious while using slippery elm bark.

Marshmallow Root (*Althaea officinalis*)

Marshmallow root helps pull excess mucus from the respiratory tract, soothes the mucous membranes of the respiratory and digestive tracts, and acts as a natural anti-inflammatory. It helps to gently eliminate waste material from the intestines. Boil one teaspoon of dried marshmallow root per cup of water for ten to fifteen minutes. Drink one cup, three times daily.

Rhubarb Root (*Rheum officinale*)

Long used by the Chinese, rhubarb root has numerous medicinal properties. It alleviates diarrhea, reduces stomach and intestinal discomfort, and promotes menstruation. It also helps loosen old fecal matter from the intestines. Boil half a teaspoon of dried root per cup of water for ten minutes. Take one tablespoon at a time, up to one cup daily. Alternatively, take quarter a teaspoon of tincture daily.

Acupressure for Intestinal Cleansing

Acupressure helps improve the flow of energy for intestinal cleansing. When I asked Donna Eden and David Feinstein, two of the foremost energy medicine experts, for the energy exercise they most recommend for intestinal cleansing, they recommended the following points. Apply firm pressure to the point and hold each point for a minute or two. You can work on both sides at the same time. For example, Stomach 36 is located below the lower and outer edges of both kneecaps. You can apply pressure to both points at the same time. To help you find the points, I have included a drawing that follows. There are two sets for each organ. The exercise is most effective if you follow the order in which they appear. Avoid Stomach 36 if you are pregnant.

Small Intestine Acupressure Points

+ Small Intestine 8(SI 8) is located just below the elbow on the back of the arm.
+ Stomach 36 (St 36) is located in the space where the two lower leg bones meet just below and to the outer edge of the kneecap.

Then:

+ Small Intestine 2 (SI 2) is located on the top of the hand about an inch above the meeting point of the ring and little fingers.
+ Urinary Bladder 66 (UB 66) is located on the outside edge of the foot, at the base of the little toe.

Large Intestine Acupressure Points:

+ Large Intestine 2 (LI 2) is located at the level of the base of the forefinger on the top of back of the hand.
+ Urinary Bladder 66 (UB 66) is located at the base of the little toe where there is a change in skin colour.

Then:

+ Large Intestine 5 (LI 5) is located in the depression found on the thumb side of the wrist.
+ Small Intestine 5 (SI 5) is located on the top of the hand at the level of the wrist, on the little finger side.

You are what you eat, digest, absorb, and assimilate. By improving your digestion and cleansing your kidneys and intestinal tracts, you'll be making big strides toward improving your overall health. Your body will thank you in the form of fewer problems with digestion, greater energy, weight normalization, and better health.

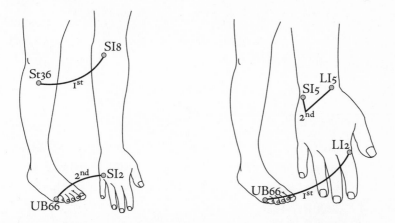

Figure 8.2 Small intestine and large intestine accupressure points.

In this chapter you learned
- The importance of the kidneys, urinary tract, and intestines to good health
- The symptoms you may be suffering indicate that the kidneys, urinary tract, and intestines may need cleansing
- How to cleanse the kidneys, urinary tract and intestines using food, herbs, and energy medicine

References

1. Ann Louise Gittleman, *The Fat Flush Plan* (New York, NY: McGraw-Hill, 2002), p. 27.

2. Michelle Schoffro Cook, "Digestion Tips That Aren't Hard to Swallow," *Natural Living* (Volume 4, Issue 4).

3. Patricia Fitzgerald, *The Detox Solution* (Santa Monica, CA: Illumination Press, 2001), p. 140.

4. Fitzgerald, *The Detox Solution*, p. 140.

5. Fitzgerald, *The Detox Solution*, p. 141.

6. Fitzgerald, *The Detox Solution*, p. 139. Jacqueline Krohn and Frances Taylor, *Natural Detoxification: A Practical Encyclopedia* (Vancouver, BC: Hartley & Marks Publishers, Inc., 2000), p. 411.

7. Adapted from Schoffro Cook, "Digestion Tips That Aren't Hard to Swallow."

8. Fitzgerald, *The Detox Solution*, p. 147.

9. Fitzgerald, *The Detox Solution*, p. 150.

10. Gittleman, *The Fat Flush Plan*, p. 24.

11. Gittleman, *The Fat Flush Plan*, p. 24.

12. Adapted from Fitzgerald, *The Detox Solution*, p. 153.

13. Gloria Gilbere, "A Doctor's Solution to 'Plumbing Problems,' In Your Gut That Is!" *Total Health*, Vol. 26, No. 1, p. 37.

14. Gilbere, "A Doctor's Solution to 'Plumbing Problems,' In Your Gut That Is!", p. 37.

15. Gilbere, "A Doctor's Solution to 'Plumbing Problems,' In Your Gut That Is!", p. 37.

CHAPTER 9

Targeting the Lymphatic System (and Cellulite)

People's natures are basically the same; it is their
practices which set them far apart.
Confucius

In this chapter you will learn
+ How the lymphatic system plays an important role in keeping your body healthy
+ The many symptoms, such as pain, inflammation, and cellulite, that are linked with a sluggish lymphatic system
+ Why it is important to cleanse your lymphatic system for optimum health
+ How to use foods, herbs, deep breathing, massage, and rebounding to assist with cleansing your lymphatic system

YOUR LYMPHATIC SYSTEM

Virtually every book on detoxification or detox program that claims to cleanse your whole body consists of cleansing two systems: the intestines and liver. The last time I looked, these two organ systems did not make up the entire human body, quite thankfully, I might add. The lymphatic system is possibly the most neglected cleansing and healing system in your body, yet it is immensely powerful.

You were introduced to the lymphatic system in Chapter 5. This system is one of the main means of efficient detoxification in your body. Mention the liver to people, and they have an idea about the organ; if you mention the lymph system to people, they may think you're speaking in tongues. Known or not, the importance of this system is undeniable. It is frequently the difference between good and poor health.

As you learned in Chapter 5, the lymph system is a complex network of fluid-filled nodes, glands, and tubes that bathe our cells and carry the body's "sewage" away from the tissues and neutralize it. A recent study found that 80 percent of overweight women have sluggish lymphatic systems and that getting them flowing smoothly is the key to easy weight loss and improved feelings of well-being.[1]

The lymphatic system comprises lymph glands, nodes, spleen, thymus, and tonsils, as well as vessels and ducts. These elements of the lymph system work together to carry cellular waste to the bloodstream. It handles toxins that enter your body from external sources such as foods or air pollution but also deals with internally produced toxins (endotoxins) that are the result of normal metabolic processes in your body. One example is inflammation in the body. The lymph system helps carry the waste products of inflammation to your blood to be eliminated.

Lymph fluid enters your veins near your heart and in doing so enters your bloodstream. Once toxins have been swept up in the lymph system and dumped into the bloodstream, the kidneys take over, filtering the blood to remove the toxins.

Lymph fluid relies on breathing, movement, and massage to flow effectively. Keeping the fluid flowing is a severe problem among most people who lead a sedentary life and breathe shallowly. However, sluggish lymph may still be an issue even if you get adequate exercise. There is three times more lymph fluid in the body than blood, yet there is no organ like the heart to pump lymph. That means it relies on deep breathing and increased activity to move.

Stress plays a role in lymph flow as well since we tend to breathe shallowly during stressful situations. During Phase 2 of the detox plan, you will begin to incorporate the deep breathing techniques discussed in Chapter 6 into your life. I encourage you to incorporate this change into your daily life even after you are finished with this plan. The benefits of improved breathing are many.

You will begin to improve the flow of the lymphatic system during *The 4-Week Ultimate Body Detox Plan*. If you are prone to problems with the lymphatic system, you may need a more concerted effort to cleanse the lymph. How do you know if your lymph system needs more cleansing? Here is a short quiz to help you decide.

The Lymph Stress Quiz

Are you overweight?

Do you have cellulite or fatty deposits?

Do you suffer from aches and pains?

Have you been diagnosed with fibromyalgia, chronic fatigue syndrome, multiple sclerosis, lupus, or other chronic immune system disorder?

Have you ever yo-yo dieted?

Do you feel bloated or have areas on your body that seem a little pudgy?

Are you prone to lumps and growths in your body?

Do you experience abdominal bloating?

Do you experience eye puffiness?

If you answered yes to any of the above questions, your lymph system could use further tuning up.

There are numerous ways to do this. You can continue with Phase 2 even after you have completed the prescribed week. Another option is to repeat Phase 2 as a stand-alone detox after you have completed the rest of the program. You can do Phase 2 for one week out of every month or for two days out of each week or you can use it to detoxify for a month at a time. Choose the approach that best fits your personality, discipline, time, and severity of your symptoms.

If you choose to use herbs for more than three weeks to assist with your lymphatic cleansing, I encourage you to consult a skilled herbalist. While using herbs to assist with lymphatic cleansing is usually quite safe, on rare occasions they can be toxic with long-term use. The human body adjusts to many circumstances, so herbs often work best when you change them periodically.

Thoroughly cleansing the lymphatic system is the key to long-term and efficient weight loss and great health. It is also the key to living without pain. The lymph system picks up toxins from your tissues and cells. If it is inefficient, then you may see fatty deposits or cellulite or experience aches and pains. Conversely, if you improve the cleansing ability of the lymph system, it will be able to "sweep" away the toxins that lead to cellulite.

A study by Dr. Elisabeth Dancey, author of *The Cellulite Solution*, found that women with cellulite showed lymphatic system deficiencies.[2] Thoroughly cleanse your lymphatic system and you will see cellulite diminish.

Ann Louise Gittleman, author of *The Fat Flush*, estimates that many people carry an extra ten to fifteen pounds of water that is trapped in their tissues, contributing to abdominal bloating, cellulite, and eye puffiness.[3] If you experience any of these symptoms or your tissues have an unnatural spongy feel to them, you may be experiencing the effects of a sluggish lymphatic system. Dr. Elson Haas, author of *The False Fat Diet*, refers to this bloating or excess fluid retention as "false fat." Many people mistakenly believe they are holding excess fat but may actually be bloated due to a sluggish lymphatic system. Ironically, if you drink inadequate amounts of water daily, your lymphatic system will slow down. It requires fluid to function properly.

A healthy lymphatic system also helps to purify your blood. One of the ways it does this is through the largest mass of lymph tissue in the body, the spleen. The spleen fights infection and destroys worn-out red blood cells in the body. It is an oval-shaped organ located to the left of the stomach. By cleansing your lymphatic system, your spleen will be better able to handle the retired red blood cells.

Cleansing the liver, in the third phase of *The 4-Week Ultimate Body Detox Plan*, also helps boost your lymphatic cleansing efforts since the liver is primarily responsible for producing lymph fluid.

Eat for a Clean Lymphatic System

Here are some of the best ways to cleanse your lymph system and get lymph fluid moving better:

Avoid chemical "foods"—that is, any foods that contain preservatives, flavours, colours, enhancers, stabilizers—in other words, most prepared, packaged, and fast foods. The farther away from the natural, whole fruit, vegetable, grain, or bean that a food has moved, the more likely it is to clog your lymphatic system.

Avoid foods that are difficult to digest, including fatty foods and simple sugars and simple carbohydrates. Most animal protein tends to be difficult to digest, requiring the body's enzymes to digest them, instead of using these enzymes for more important functions. Sweet foods and the "whites," which include white rice, white bread, white pasta, and any white flour products, require enormous amounts of energy to handle the resulting rapid blood sugar fluctuations. This energy is better served to cleanse your lymph.

Drink plenty of water—as mentioned above, without adequate water, lymph fluid cannot flow properly. Lymph is a liquid and therefore requires water to flow. What if you totally stopped watering your plants? They would not survive. At first they might get a few brown spots or yellow leaves, then leaves would turn brown and fall off, and eventually the whole plant would become crisp and die. Plants need water to live. We are the same. Our bodies, including our lymph systems, need water to function properly. Like plants, some things would begin to deteriorate, then more systems in our bodies would fail, and eventually we would die without adequate water. Few of us consider our inadequate water intake as a source of our pain, discomfort, or other health problems. Forget the soda, trash the colour-laden sports drinks, and drop the sugary fruit punch. As Dr. Phil would say, it's time to "get real." Drink real water—the very stuff your cells depend on for health.

The enzymes and acids in raw fruit are powerful lymph cleansers, particularly when eaten on an empty stomach. That is one of the reasons you eat raw fruit in the morning on *The 4-Week Ultimate Body Detox Plan*. Add more raw fruits, vegetables, salads, and fresh juices to your diet, and your lymph will have the tools it needs to do some serious deep cleansing.

Flavonoids, malic acid, citric acid, quinic acid, and enzymes (only in raw cranberries, not in pasteurised bottled cranberry juice) in cranberries and cranberry juice help to emulsify stubborn fat in the lymphatic system. Be sure to drink only pure, unsweetened cranberry juice. Dilute it about 4:1 water to cranberry juice. Alternatively, if you prefer a less tart juice, dilute one part unsweetened cranberry juice with two parts pure apple juice and two parts water. Make sure you use only pure apple juice devoid of sweeteners or preservatives.

Eat plenty of green vegetables to provide chlorophyll (the green colour in plants) and loads of vitamins and minerals to assist in lymph cleansing.

Flax seeds and flax oil contain essential fatty acids that are required by your body for most functions, including lymphatic system functions. Grind flax seeds in a coffee grinder and sprinkle them on bread, grains, fruit, soy yogurt, or other food. Do not cook flax seeds. After grinding them, keep flax seeds covered in the refrigerator. Use cold-pressed flax oil on salads or pour it on steamed vegetables or baked potatoes. Again, do not heat flax oil. Simply pour on food after it has been cooked. Try to consume at least one to two tablespoons of flax oil and two tablespoons of ground flax seeds daily.

Organic eggs are helpful during lymphatic system cleansing. They provide a useable form of protein that prevents fluid from flowing into the spaces between cells. If fluid becomes trapped in these spaces due to insufficient protein intake, your body will hold onto excess water, may become bloated, and gain water weight. Eat only organic eggs, however, since other kinds typically contain synthetic hormones and antibiotics that are given to hens to supposedly prevent disease and stimulate egg production. These items do not belong in your body and can disrupt your body's own hormone and intestinal bacteria balance. Restrict your consumption to several organic eggs per week.

Avoid large, heavy meals. Instead, eat smaller meals and snack between meals. Eat only when you are hungry, not when you are bored. If you are bored, find something else to do.

Foods high in essential fatty acids are critical to ensure a properly functioning lymph system. Some of these foods include fresh raw walnuts, almonds, hazelnuts, macadamias, Brazil nuts, and other types of nuts; sunflower seeds, flax seeds, and pumpkin seeds; avocadoes; and cold-pressed oils. Be sure to eat fresh raw nuts and seeds that can be found in the refrigerator section of your local health food or grocery store. The essential fatty acids found in nuts and seeds go rancid easily. Eating rancid nuts and seeds exposes your body to further toxins that attack and damage cells. Eating fresh raw nuts and seeds provides your body with essential building blocks for health and life. In addition, they taste better.

The enzyme protease is helpful for moving lymph since it breaks down many toxins that have a protein coating. Protease helps break down bacteria, viruses, cancer cells, and inflammation in the body. Protease is found in raw nuts, seeds, and fruits and vegetables, particularly those that have a higher protein content. Nature is truly miraculous. It supplies protein and the enzymes needed to digest protein, provided the foods are not heated above 118 degrees F (since all enzymes are destroyed above that temperature).

Clean Up Your Lymph

In addition to eating well to cleanse your lymphatic system, there are many other things you can do to get and keep your lymph moving freely. Here are some of the things you can do:

Try to get adequate sleep since sleep helps eliminate stress hormones from the body. These hormones encourage fat storage and a sluggish lymphatic system.

Studies show that virtually any type of massage can push up to 78 percent of stagnant lymph back into circulation. Massage frees trapped toxins. Follow the massage suggested in Chapter 6 to encourage lymphatic cleansing. In addition, you may wish to see a massage therapist skilled at lymphatic drainage massage. Lymphatic drainage is a specific form of massage that helps to encourage lymph flow and often works even with the most stubborn cases of fluid buildup.

Essential oils such as geranium, juniper, and black pepper can be used in a bath or diluted in a pure oil as a body oil to stimulate the lymphatic system through massage and improve the flow of lymph, thereby helping your body eliminate toxins. See Chapter 6 for more details about using these oils to stimulate lymph cleansing.

Dry skin brushing helps improve lymphatic circulation. It is a simple practice that requires about a minute or two per day. Follow the instructions mentioned in Chapter 6.

Stretching and aerobic types of exercise stimulate the lymphatic system to help lymph flow. These include yoga, walking, Pilates, and, of course, rebounding. Rebounding on a mini trampoline forces the millions of one-way valves in the lymphatic system to open, increasing lymph flow up to fourteen times, according to Morton Walker, author of *Jumping for Health*. Learn more about rebounding in Chapter 6.

Deep breathing creates muscular contractions and movement. The added oxygen also helps pump lymphatic fluid. You learned some powerful breathing exercises in Chapter 6 that help move lymph fluid.

Stagnant lymph increases the toxic load in the body. This can affect memory and mental function and contribute to inflammation, pain, and bloating. It can result in cellulite, fatty deposits, and disorders such as fibromyalgia and chronic fatigue syndrome, among others.

Alternating hot and cold showers helps to stimulate lymph flow in the body. I have included a hydrotherapy treatment in Chapter 6. It is an excellent adjunct therapy to incorporate into your lymph cleansing for optimum results. You can also use it any time you want a boost in your blood circulation. Be sure to check with your physician if you suspect any heart or blood pressure problems or have other medical concerns before attempting this hydrotherapy treatment.

Herbs for Deep Lymphatic Cleansing

There are many excellent herbs that help with lymphatic cleansing, including echinacea, astragalus, cleavers, goldenseal, pokeroot, and wild indigo root. If you are pregnant or have a serious health condition, consult a medical doctor before using any herbs. Consult a herbalist before combining two or more herbs or while taking medication with herbs. Avoid long-term use of any herb (longer than three weeks) without first consulting a qualified herbalist.

Echinacea (*Echinacea, various species*)

Based on echinacea's current popularity, it may be hard to imagine that over the last century echinacea was reviled. This powerful lymphatic system cleanser has a proven track record for its ability to increase the body's immune response. Combined with another good lymph cleanser, astragalus, echinacea helps to reduce congestion and swelling. Make a decoction using two teaspoons of dried herb per cup of water. Bring to a boil. Simmer for fifteen minutes. Drink one cup, three times a day. Alternatively, take one teaspoon of tincture, three times a day.

Astragalus (*Astragalus, various species*)

Astragalus is an excellent lymphatic system cleanser and liver protector. It works well, especially when combined with echinacea, to alleviate congestion and swelling in the body. The Chinese have been using astragalus, which they refer to as "huang qi" for over two thousand years. Huang qi means life force strengthener. Astragalus is primarily available as a tincture or in capsule or tablet form. Since potency can vary greatly with this herb, it is best to follow the package directions for the optimum dose.

Cleavers (*Galium aparine, also known as Goosegrass or Grip Grass*)

The green parts of the plant are used (stems and small leaves). Cleavers cleanses the blood, is an anti-inflammatory, decreases the body's tendency to form tumours, increases urinary flow, and tones and strengthens the body, all while enhancing the function of the lymphatic system. It is an excellent herb for swollen glands and swollen tonsils. Cleavers improves the ability of the lymphatic system to deal with toxins. It combines well with another herb, pokeroot. For cleavers tea, use two to three teaspoons of the dried herb per cup of water. Drink one cup three times daily. Alternatively use a half to one teaspoon of tincture three times a day. Avoid using cleavers if you suffer from diabetes or have diabetic tendencies.

Goldenseal (*Hydrastis canadensis*)

In addition to having anti-inflammatory properties, goldenseal helps to break down excess catarrh in the lungs, kills parasites, decreases pain, has laxative properties, stimulates muscles and digestion, tones and strengthens the skin and mucous membranes, and encourages lymphatic cleansing. Use a half to one teaspoon of dried herb per cup for an infusion. You can drink this mixture or use it as a wash. Alternatively take a half to one teaspoon of tincture three times a day.

Pokeroot (*Phytolacca americana*)

Pokeroot is a useful herb for improving the flow of lymph. It works well with immune- and lymph-related conditions such as adenitis, tonsillitis, laryngitis, swollen glands, mumps, mastitis, and fibrocystic breast disease. Pokeroot helps to break down excess mucus in the body, eases rheumatic pain, is a strong laxative, and is an overall stimulant. It combines well with blue flag. Take one-third teaspoon per cup and simmer for fifteen minutes as a decoction. Alternatively, take one-eighth to one-quarter teaspoon of the tincture, three times a day. Do not increase the dose. The powerful laxative effects of this herb can be harmful in larger doses.

Wild Indigo Root (*Baptisia tinctoria*)

The root of the wild indigo plant helps destroy damaging microbes in the body, breaks down excess mucus and catarrh, decreases fevers, and of course, cleans up the lymphatic system and improves lymph flow. It works well if you have mucous congestion due to consuming dairy products or if you have acute reactions to eating dairy products. You can probably guess then that it is beneficial for the nose, sinuses, ears, and throat. It is helpful for conditions such as laryngitis, pharyngitis, tonsillitis, swollen lymph glands, and fevers. If infections are present in these areas of the body, it is helpful to combine wild indigo root with echinacea. For lymphatic problems, it combines well with cleavers and pokeroot. You can take it as a decoction using one-third teaspoon of the dried root per cup of water. Simmer fifteen minutes. Take one cup three times a day. Alternatively, take a quarter to a half teaspoon of tincture three times per day.

Supercharge Your Lymph Cleansing Efforts

Donna Eden and David Feinstein recommend vigorously massaging any of the following areas wherever there is tenderness to encourage the flow of energy in areas where there are many lymphatic vessels or nodes. The following diagrams illustrate the neurolymphatic massage points suggested by Eden and Feinstein. The sorer the area, the more in need of massage it may be. This massage can take place anywhere, even while clothed. You do not need to be undressed to take a minute or two to vigorously rub any neurolymphatic massage points that feel tender.

In this chapter you learned
- How the lymphatic system plays an important role in keeping your body healthy
- That many common symptoms like pain, inflammation, and cellulite are signs of a sluggish lymphatic system
- That you must cleanse your lymphatic system for optimum health
- How to use foods, herbs, deep breathing, massage, and rebounding to assist with cleansing your lymphatic system

References

1. Jillian Boyle, "Is Lymphatic Stress the Reason You're Fat? Bloated? Hungry for Junk Food?" *Woman's World*, March 2, 2004.

2. Ann Louise Gittleman, *The Fat Flush Plan* (McGraw-Hill, New York: 2002), p. 21.

3. Gittleman, *The Fat Flush Plan*, p. 20.

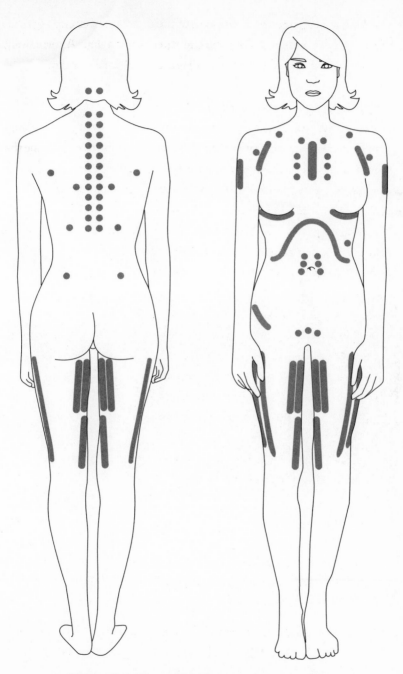

Figure 9.1 Neurolymphatic massage points

CHAPTER 10

Targeting the Liver and Gallbladder

"Healing is a matter of time, but it is sometimes
also a matter of opportunity."
Hippocrates

In this chapter you will learn
+ The many important functions of the gallbladder and liver
+ The symptoms and disorders linked with an unhealthy liver and gallbladder
+ Why it is imperative to great health to cleanse your liver and gallbladder
+ How to use foods, herbs, and energy medicine to assist with your liver and gallbladder detoxification

YOUR LIVER

Your liver has over five hundred different functions, making it one of the most overworked organs in your body. A few of these functions include storing certain vitamins, minerals, and sugars for use as fuel; controlling both the production and excretion of cholesterol; and creating the thousands of enzymes that control virtually every function of your body. The liver also secretes a substance called bile that is stored in the gallbladder. You'll learn a bit more about bile when we discuss the valuable role of the gallbladder below. The liver metabolizes proteins, fats, and carbohydrates and processes hemoglobin in the blood to allow use of its iron. The liver controls the production and excretion of cholesterol in your body. Literally, the liver performs more biochemical tasks than any other organ in your body.

The liver is a particularly stressed organ as a direct result of our modern lifestyle. All foreign substances that enter your body have to be filtered by your liver. These include alcohol; tobacco; environmental pollutants; food additives; pesticides; common cosmetic ingredients; household products; stress or excess sex hormones; thyroid or adrenal hormones; pharmaceutical and over-the-counter (OTC) drugs; caffeine; and much more.

You recently learned that the average person consumes fourteen pounds of food preservatives, additives, waxes, colourings, flavours, antimicrobials, and pesticide residues per year.[1] Your liver is responsible for filtering all of these chemicals and many more. The liver must filter medications, including commonly used antibiotics and acetaminophen, sometimes resulting in damage to this important organ. It is critical in our modern age of chemical exposure to keep your liver functioning as efficiently as possible.

The liver breaks fat-soluble chemicals into water-soluble compounds to prevent the body from storing these toxins in fat. This takes place in Phase 1 of detoxification in the liver. This phase begins the process of detoxifying substances such as car exhaust, medications, and internally produced substances such as hormones. In the second phase of liver detoxification, the liver breaks down toxins to convert them into harmless waste products that can be expelled via the urine or stool.

As I've said, many people dive head-over-heels into liver cleansing (and many health practitioners suggest this approach) but it can be damaging to a person if their kidneys and intestines are not prepared for increased toxin elimination. That is one of the reasons why it is imperative to cleanse the kidneys and intestines before beginning liver detoxification. The toxins can build up in the liver, like a dam, then get dumped into the urinary and intestinal tract where they are unable to be released and get further backed up, resulting in damage to the body.

It is also imperative that both phases of liver detoxification are functioning optimally and at the same pace. If either phase is sluggish, the liver cannot keep pace with toxins that enter the body. Toxins will continue to circulate through the blood and add extra burden to the other detox organs. The other detox organs are not capable of handling the liver's job. This is like the engineering department attempting to do the job of the accounting department in an organization. They may be able to do some of the work, but more likely they do not have the training or skills to handle all the functions. An accounting backlog will ensue.

When the liver cannot handle all the toxins thrown at it and toxins continue to circulate through the body, you may begin to experience uncomfortable symptoms—the signs of an overburdened liver, which is also known as liver toxicity.

Dr. Scott Rigden conducted a study of over two hundred patients suffering from chronic fatigue syndrome and/or fibromyalgia. He found that 80 percent of all sufferers of these two disorders had significant liver impairment. As patients' symptoms improved, so did the results of liver function tests—indicating a correlation between liver stress and severity of symptoms of chronic fatigue syndrome and fibromyalgia.[2]

Detoxification of the liver, in its simplest terms, is divided into two phases, aptly named Phase 1 and Phase 2. Either or both phases can be hindered by toxic buildup in the body. Toxins initially enter the liver in Phase 1, during which time they are broken down into smaller fragments to allow easier elimination. Then they pass to Phase 2 in the liver, where enzymes convert toxins to more water-soluble forms or molecules (such as glutathione, glycine, and sulfate) are added to toxins to create substances that are less toxic to the body so they can be eliminated in the bile, urine, or stool.

Phase 1 can be hindered if too many toxins enter the liver at once. Phase 2 can often be inefficient at keeping up with the toxins leaving Phase 1, thereby creating an imbalance that often results in symptoms of drug or environmental chemical intolerances. In such cases, people may have trouble with perfumes (after all, they are mostly made up of synthetic and toxic chemicals), gas fumes, paint, or other chemicals.

If the liver is overloaded with toxins, these toxins can leave the liver to be stored in fat tissue, central nervous system cells, and your brain. These stored toxins may circulate in the blood at other times, contributing to chronic disease. Inefficient detoxification in the liver is suspected by holistic health experts to play a role in many diseases, including skin disorders, arthritis, chronic fatigue syndrome, fibromyalgia, and inflammation in the body.

The liver simply was not designed to handle all the synthetic chemicals in modern life. In the past one hundred years, the liver has become increasingly abused through exposure to chemicalized and processed foods, pharmaceutical drugs, chemically treated water, vehicle exhaust, chemical cleaners, and hydrogenated oils and trans fats. Hydrogenated oils are foreigners to the body. They are artificially hardened using metal and hydrogen gas. Eating them is comparable to eating plastic food and almost as toxic. Manufacturers of many "fake fats" such as margarine—a fat that is supposed to go through your body undigested—do not have even a modest interest in the workings of the body. They prey on people who believe that these fake fats will travel from the mouth to the colon untouched. The body does not work that way. The main organ that is compromised by these toxic fats is the liver. It will become clogged and inefficient at its job. You will likely start to gain weight or suffer skin problems or have headaches or some other unwanted problem by continuing to abuse the liver.

Many people choose to eat a low-fat diet despite what researchers and nutritionists have been claiming for years. Eating a low-fat diet will result in deficiencies of essential fatty acids, which are needed for a healthy body. On such a diet, your body will have symptoms of fatty acid deficiencies, usually in four weeks or less. One of the most common symptoms is a slowed metabolism. The liver also slows, making it less efficient at breaking down fat in the body as well as the many toxins it is exposed to. That means more toxic substances circulating throughout the body. I cringe when I hear someone tell me that they eat a "good, low-fat diet to lose weight." You will not lose weight on a low-fat diet. More likely you will gain numerous health problems.

The liver simply cannot handle the onslaught of synthetic chemicals we throw at it. Yet even when the liver has lost up to 80 percent of its ability to function, it continues working. But working and working optimally are two substantially different things. We are interested in improving the liver's function so that it works optimally.

Perhaps the most impressive thing about the liver is its ability to regenerate itself. When it is given the critical nutrients, a healthy non-stressful diet, and herbs to help it function, it can be restored to health in most circumstances.

GALLBLADDER

Your gallbladder is a small organ that sits below the liver on the right side of your abdomen, under the rib cage. Through a series of ducts, it is connected to the liver and the small intestines. The gallbladder secretes a green-coloured substance called bile to help break down fat and stimulate contractions of the intestines to push waste matter out of your bowels. The liver produces bile and sends it to the gallbladder for storage and secretion as necessary. Most bile is circulated in the digestive tract. If the waste matter in the intestines is not moving through at a healthy speed, bile may be reabsorbed through the walls of the intestine and returned to the liver in the bloodstream.

Some of the symptoms that are associated with gallbladder toxicity include difficulty digesting fatty foods, skin problems, migraines, joint problems, chronic neck problems, pain in the upper abdomen (usually lasting twenty minutes to several hours), pain between the shoulder blades, nausea, vomiting, or any symptoms that worsen after eating fatty foods. Even heart problems are sometimes linked to gallbladder toxicity when the gallbladder is not adequately controlling blood fats.

Of course, there is also the concern about gallstones. Gallstones are solid pieces of crystalline material that form when the gallbladder does not secrete adequate bile over time. They range in size from a grain of sand to a golf ball and are made up of fats, cholesterol, bile pigments, and minerals in bile. About 80 percent of all gallstones, according to some estimates, are made of cholesterol and are typically white or yellowish-coloured. Other stones are darker and are made up of calcium salts and an orangey-yellow waste product in the body called bilirubin. Bilirubin is what gives urine its yellow colour.

Over one million people in the United States are diagnosed with gallstones every year. While in theory the gallbladder should be able to keep up with the body's toxin load, this is often not the case, particularly in people who eat a fatty diet over long periods of time (i.e., the average person in North America), take birth control pills or hormone replacement therapy, smoke cigarettes, drink heavily, go on crash diets or lose weight quickly, or eat a low-fibre diet with lots of sugary or starchy foods (also the average North American). Pregnancy, diabetes, pancreatitis, obesity, and celiac disease are also factors that may increase the risk of gallbladder toxicity.

Liver and Gallbladder Stress Quiz

Do you suffer from any of the following signs of liver toxicity?[3]

Abdominal bloating
Alcohol intolerance
Allergies
Arthritis (some types)
Asthma
Bad breath or a coated tongue
Bowel infections
Brain "fog"
Chronic fatigue syndrome
Crohn's disease
Cravings for sweets
Dark circles under the eyes
Depression
Difficulty losing weight
Environmental illness or multiple chemical sensitivities
Fatigue
Fatty liver
Fevers
Fibromyalgia
Fluid retention
Gallbladder disease
Gallstones or gravel

Gastritis

Headaches and migraines

Hepatitis

High blood pressure

High cholesterol levels

Hives

Hypoglycemia (unstable blood sugar levels)

Hormone imbalances

Immune system disorders

Indigestion

Irritable bowel syndrome

Mood swings

Overweight or obesity

Poor appetite

Poor digestion

Recurring nausea and/or vomiting with no known cause

Skin diseases

Slow metabolism

Ulcerative colitis

If you are suffering from any of these symptoms, you may benefit from further cleansing of your liver and gallbladder, which will in turn strengthen your body's ability to break down fat and fatty deposits.

Eat for a Clean Liver and Gallbladder

Your intestinal tract should be functioning optimally before cleansing the liver. That means you should be having two to three large bowel movements daily, typically after each time you eat.

Eating a healthy diet is imperative for optimal liver functioning. The liver requires high amounts of vitamins and minerals to perform its many functions. Your diet should be high in fruits and vegetables and fibre-rich foods. It should be free of processed foods, artificial food additives, colours, preservatives, and animal foods such as meat, poultry, and dairy products. A diet low in refined sugar and fatty foods is important as well. Avoid synthetic sweeteners. Try to eat foods that are devoid of pesticides and synthetic chemicals used in the growing processes. Avoid drinking with meals. Drink just enough water at mealtimes to take nutritional or herbal supplements. Avoid eating if you feel particularly stressed or anxiety-ridden.

Eat only when you are hungry and stop when you are full. Eating fruit in the morning is helpful for liver cleansing, as is eating a large, raw salad with lunch and dinner. Conversely, if you are hungry, eat. Too many people literally starve themselves and their bodies of adequate nutrition because they refrain from eating throughout the day. Your body needs proper nourishment to work properly. Remember the car analogy I used earlier?

As with cleansing any of the other organ systems, you will need to drink between eight and ten glasses of pure, filtered water every day. This is the only way to flush toxins out of your body. Your cells require fluid to work properly and to suspend toxins for elimination. A recent study showed a higher incidence of Alzheimer's disease in people who do not drink enough water.[4]

During *The 4-Week Ultimate Body Detox Plan*, you start every morning with lemon water. This is a great practice to continue whenever you wish to cleanse your liver. In addition, taking one to three tablespoons of pectin in water or pure fruit juice helps to absorb toxins. Eat a couple of apples per day to obtain the pectin they contain.

Eat at least two carrots per day (baby carrots don't count as a full carrot) and one or more beets every day, both of which are powerful liver-cleansing and rebuilding foods. In addition, eat two large green salads or a minimum of one cup of green veggies per day. The chlorophyll that gives plants their green colour, helps cleanse the liver.

Try to eat two heaping tablespoons of ground flax seeds. They bind to hormone receptor sites, preventing excess hormones from floating around your bloodstream. One of the liver's five hundred jobs is to filter excess hormones. By eating flax seeds and flax oil you are helping it function more effectively. Flaxseeds can be sprinkled on cereal, toast, salads, or blended into smoothies.

Include one to two tablespoons of cold-pressed flax seed oil into your diet to help cleanse the liver and gallbladder. Actually, this is an excellent practice to maintain even after you have finished your cleanse. Flax seed oil provides essential fatty acids that are critical to keep your liver functioning optimally, in addition to their many other uses within the body.

Research shows consuming seven to ten servings of fruit and vegetables per day helps people lose more weight than cutting back on sugary and fatty foods. Evidence also confirms that high produce consumption cuts your risk of getting *all* types of cancer and lowers the risk of getting heart disease by 40 percent.[5]

Eat one or two cloves of garlic, the equivalent of one-half onion (this can be part of an entrée that incorporates the onion for flavour), and a handful of broccoli spears per day, since these foods contain sulphur, which is required to increase enzyme activity (and therefore increase liver cleansing activity).

Avoid eating large meals. Instead, eat small meals made up of plenty of easy-to-digest foods. Eat steamed vegetables, raw salad greens, raw fruits, and bitter greens. The bitter greens help to stimulate bile flow. Eat whole, raw, unsalted nuts and seeds for their essential fatty acids as well as their usable protein.

Avoid eating heavy, fatty foods since they just create more work for the liver and optimum conditions for the formation of gallstones. You should definitely be avoiding margarine, shortening, commercial oils and any foods made with them. Avoid eating animal fat and fried foods as well.

Avoid eating refined carbohydrates such as white bread, pastries, cookies, cakes, white pasta, white sugar, and soft drinks. Avoid coffee, chocolate, and spicy foods while cleansing the liver.

If you are suffering from gallstones or a sluggish gallbladder, drink three to four cups of pure unsweetened apple juice daily. The malic acid in the juice helps to break down stones and stagnant bile.

If you have difficulty with the vegetarian nature of this program, you may wish to eat organic eggs in moderation while cleansing the liver and gallbladder. They contain lecithin, which is needed for liver cleansing. Soybeans, tofu, soy milk, and other soy foods also contain lecithin.

Avoid eating for several hours before bedtime to allow the liver adequate time during the night to perform its many functions, unimpeded by other bodily processes.

FOODS THAT BURN FAT

The liver is the primary organ to help your body metabolize fat. If you are overweight or have a few extra bulges you'd be happy to be rid of, you can increase the fat-burning power of the detoxification by adding more foods that help your liver to burn fat better. There are many fabulous foods that fight fat, but the ones below are my picks as the top twelve.

Top 12 Fat-Fighting Foods

1. **Oatmeal:** This complex carbohydrate (the good kind) is slow to digest and helps to keep blood sugar levels stable while keeping you feeling full. Research also shows that consuming oatmeal reduces a person's cravings for fatty foods.[6] Be sure to eat the unsweetened kind.
2. **Leafy Greens:** Spinach, spring mix, mustard greens, and other dark leafy greens are good sources of fibre and power-houses of nutrition. Research demonstrates that their high concentration of vitamins and antioxidants helps prevent hunger while protecting you from heart disease, cancer, cataracts, and memory loss.[7]

3. **Olives and Olive Oil**: Being rich in healthy fats, olives and olive oil help to reduce cravings for junky foods and keep you feeling full. Research shows that monounsaturated fats that are plentiful in these foods help reduce high blood pressure.[8]

4. **Beans and Legumes**: Legumes are the best source of fibre of any foods. They help to stabilize blood sugar while keeping you regular. They are also high in potassium, a critical mineral that reduces dehydration and the risk of high blood pressure and stroke. A legume, soy is particularly good for fat-burning. Isoflavones found in soy foods speed the breakdown of stored fat. In one study, those who consumed high amounts of soy products shed three times more superfluous weight than did their counterparts who ate no soy.[9]

5. and 6. **Garlic and Onions**: These yummy foods contain phytochemicals that break down fatty deposits in the body, while also breaking down cholesterol; killing viruses, bacteria, and fungi; and protecting against heart disease.[10]

7. **Tomatoes**: Packed with vitamin C and the phytochemical lycopene, tomatoes stimulate the production of the amino acid known as carnitine. Research has shown that carnitine helps speed the body's fat-burning capacity by one-third. Lycopene is a powerful antioxidant that studies show cuts the risk of heart disease by 29 percent.[11]

8. **Nuts**: Raw, unsalted nuts provide your body with essential fatty acids that help burn fat. Their high nutrient content also lowers the risk of heart attack by 60 percent. Research shows that consuming nuts can be as effective as cholesterol-lowering drugs to reduce high cholesterol levels, not to mention they taste better and have no nasty side effects.[12]

9. **Cayenne**: This hot spice lowers the risk of excess insulin in the body by speeding metabolism and lowering blood glucose (sugar) levels, before the excess insulin can result in fat stores.[13]

10. **Turmeric:** The popular spice used primarily in Indian cooking contains the highest known source of beta carotene, the antioxidant that helps protect the liver from free radical damage. Turmeric also helps your liver heal (see below) while helping your body metabolize fats by decreasing the fat storage rate in liver cells.[14]

11. **Cinnamon:** Researchers at the United States Department of Agriculture showed that a one-quarter to one teaspoon of cinnamon with food helps metabolize sugar up to twenty times better than food not eaten with cinnamon.[15] Excess sugar in the blood can lead to fat storage.

12. **Flax Seeds and Flax Seed Oil:** These seeds and oil attract oil-soluble toxins that are lodged in the fatty tissues of the body to escort them out.[16]

Nutrients for Improving Liver and Gallbladder Function

Take one or two digestive enzyme tablets with every meal. Ideally, the tablet should include the following: proteases I, II, and III, maltase, amylase, lipase, cellulase, peptidase, lactase, and invertase.

For optimal liver cleansing, take two tablespoons of high-quality, cold-pressed flax seed oil as part of your diet. In addition, add one to two tablespoons of freshly ground (use a small coffee grinder) flax seeds, sprinkled on food, after it has been cooked. Avoid cooking flax seeds or flax oil.

Eat plenty of garlic and onions since they are high in sulphur, which is important to help your liver function optimally. In addition, eat plenty of the other top twelve fat-fighting foods mentioned above.

Lecithin helps the liver metabolize fats and reduce cholesterol. It contains a substance called phosphatidylcholine and essential fatty acids that help keep liver cells healthy and help prevent fatty deposits from building up in the liver. Lecithin also helps reduce high blood pressure by allowing the blood vessels to relax to allow better blood flow. You can get lecithin in soy foods such as soy milk, tofu, and miso, as well as organic eggs. Alternatively, take 4000 mg of lecithin in capsule form daily.

Take a high-quality multivitamin and mineral supplement. In addition, take 1000 to 3000 mg of vitamin C daily, even if there is vitamin C in your multivitamin.

The amino acid taurine is needed for liver support, especially for liver-related disorders in which tissues swell or fluid accumulates. Taurine helps your liver manufacture bile and metabolize fats and break down cholesterol. Taurine is required to keep bile fluid and to remove toxic chemicals from the body.

Clean Up Your Liver and Gallbladder

For people who are very ill and show signs of severe toxicity or are aware of extreme toxic exposure, cleansing the liver should be done slowly and gradually over months for best results. Consult a holistic doctor if you suspect liver or gallbladder disease.

Avoid use of acetominophen (Tylenol and similar painkillers) since it destroys glutathione in the liver, particularly when combined with alcohol. Refrain from consuming alcohol while cleansing and rebuilding your liver since all alcohol must be filtered by the liver and adds undue stress to a potentially stressed organ. Avoid taking any medications not prescribed by a doctor.

It is important to exercise regularly while cleansing your liver to increase the oxygen available for enzyme production and therefore liver and gallbladder detoxification. Before breakfast is the ideal time to exercise while conducting a liver and gallbladder cleanse.

While lying flat on your back, you can gently massage the liver-gallbladder area, which is located along the lower rib area on the right side of your body. This helps improve circulation to the area.

Herbs for Deep Liver and Gallbladder Cleansing

There are many powerful herbs that help with liver and gallbladder cleansing, while helping to heal both organs. Some of the best ones include milk thistle, dandelion root, globe artichoke, turmeric, slippery elm, greater celandine, balmony, barberry, black root, blue flag, boldo, fringetree bark, vervain, and wahoo. If you are pregnant or have a serious health condition, consult a medical doctor before using any herbs. Consult an herbalist before combining two or more herbs or if you are taking medication with herbs. Avoid long-term use of any herb (longer than three weeks) without first consulting a qualified herbalist.

Milk Thistle (*Silybum marianum*)

The primary medicinal ingredient in milk thistle is called silymarin. This compound protects the liver by inhibiting damaging substances in the liver that cause liver cell damage. Silymarin also stimulates liver cell regeneration to help the liver rebuild after it has been damaged.[17] Silymarin also helps to prevent the depletion of the nutrient glutathione—one of the most critical nutrients for liver detoxification. Alcohol consumption and many synthetic chemicals deplete glutathione in the liver.

Milk thistle is one of the most well-researched liver herbs. With more than one hundred studies that successfully demonstrate milk thistle's liver-protecting and -regenerating properties,[18] milk thistle makes an excellent choice for cleansing and rebuilding the liver. Milk thistle has proven itself helpful for hepatitis, cirrhosis, liver damage, cholestasis (bile stagnation), and alcohol- and chemical-induced fatty liver. Silymarin also stimulates hepatocytes (liver cells) to replace diseased tissue. A one-month study involving 129 patients showed that milk thistle brought a 50 percent improvement in the symptoms of toxic-metabolic liver damage, fatty degeneration of the liver, liver enlargement, and chronic hepatitis.[19]

Another ingredient in milk thistle, silybin, is believed to protect the genetic material within the liver cells, thereby improving the synthesis of proteins in the liver and reducing the risk of liver cancer.[20] Milk thistle aids in soothing the mucous membranes, which is helpful if gallstones or inflammation of the gallbladder is present.

Milk thistle increases liver enzyme production, repairs damaged liver tissue, and blocks the damaging effects of some toxins.[21] Over one hundred studies show the liver-supporting properties of the active ingredient, silymarin.[22]

In one study silymarin, extracted from milk thistle, protected the livers of animals that were given large doses of the common painkiller acetaminophen from damage. In another study, silymarin minimized the damage from long-term exposure to several toxic industrial chemicals, including toluene (commonly found in nail polish) and xylene. Initially, workers had abnormal levels of liver enzymes, indicating damage. After taking 140 mg of silymarin, three times per day, their liver enzymes normalized.

Silymarin in milk thistle seeds is not very water-soluble so does not extract well into tea. Instead, take a standardized extract containing about 140 mg of silymarin for liver cleansing and protection.

Dandelion Root (*Taraxacum officinale*)

Nature grows a liver-cleansing pharmacy every spring. It is the dreaded weed that most people curse as it pokes its yellow-flowered head through the green of their lawn. Dandelion is one of Mother Nature's finest liver herbs.

You already learned that dandelion has cleansing effects on the kidneys and urinary tract, but it is also a superb cleansing herb for the liver. It helps to clear obstructions and stimulate the liver to eliminate toxins. It also helps stimulate bile flow from the liver, which is important to release toxins and prevent clogging of the liver. The *Australian Journal of Medical Herbalism* cited two studies that showed the liver-regenerating properties of dandelion in cases of jaundice, liver swelling, hepatitis, and indigestion.[23] Dandelion is also helpful as a laxative and anti-inflammatory herb. It stimulates the gallbladder to encourage the flow of bile and the normal digestion of fats. It reduces the risk of gallstones. Dandelion also reduces the symptoms of arthritis and rheumatism. It works well combined with milk thistle or bayberry.

According to Ann Louise Gittleman, author of *The Fat Flush Plan*, dandelion root aids the liver and fat metabolism in two ways: it stimulates the liver to produce more bile to send to the gallbladder, and at the same time causes the gallbladder to contract and release its stored bile, assisting with fat metabolism.[24]

If you choose to incorporate dandelion root into your liver cleansing efforts, take 500 to 2000 mg daily in capsules. Alternatively, you can make a decoction by using two teaspoons of powdered dandelion root per cup of water. Bring to a boil and simmer for fifteen minutes. Drink one cup, three times daily. A third option is to take one teaspoon of the tincture, three times daily.

Globe Artichoke (*Cynara scolymus*)
Globe artichoke contains compounds called caffeylquinic acids, which have demonstrated powerful liver-regenerating effects similar to those of milk thistle.[25] Substantial research shows its capacity to protect and regenerate the liver and clean the blood. It has been helpful in cases of liver insufficiency, liver damage, liver diseases, poor digestion, gallstones, and chronic constipation. It has also helped lower cholesterol and triglycerides. Globe artichoke is usually found in capsule form. Doses range from 300 to 500 mg daily.

Turmeric (*Curcuma longal*)
A commonly used spice in Indian curries, turmeric helps regenerate liver cells and cleanse the liver of toxins. Turmeric also increases the

production of bile to help expel toxins and may help reduce liver in-flammation. Turmeric has also been shown to increase levels of two liver-supporting enzymes that promote Phase 2 liver detoxification reactions. Turmeric is also great for decreasing cholesterol levels and for decreasing pain and inflammation in other parts of the body. There are numerous ways to benefit from the healing properties of turmeric. You can mix equal parts of turmeric and honey to form a paste and take it by the teaspoonful, up to five teaspoons per day. A word of warning: your teeth may temporarily turn a yellowish colour, so be sure to keep a toothbrush nearby. Turmeric also comes in capsules and tablets, some-times under the label "curcumin," which is the key ingredient in turmeric. You can follow the Indian lead and cook with turmeric to create some delicious curry dishes. You will find a recipe for Lentil Dahl in Chapter 13 that uses turmeric. James Duke, one of the foremost herbal experts, recommends the following tea combination for the liver in his book *The Green Pharmacy*. Mix to taste: licorice, dandelion, chicory, turmeric, and ginger. Store in a jar and use one teaspoonful of herb per cup of boiling water to make a tea. Drink one cup, three times daily.

Slippery Elm (*Ulmus fulva or Ulmus campestris*)
Slippery elm bark is good for problems with the mucous membranes of the digestive tract, such as gastritis and stomach ulcers. People with severely toxic livers and abnormal bile production sometimes suffer from irritations of the mucous membranes. Make a decoction of slippery elm bark using two teaspoons of dried herb per cup of water. Drink one cup, three times daily. Alternatively, take one tea-spoon of the tincture, three times daily. If you are prone to allergies, be cautious while using slippery elm bark.

Greater Celandine (*Chelidonium majus*)
All parts of this plant—roots, stems, leaves, and flowers—offer me-dicinal properties that are helpful for cleansing the liver, urinary

tract, intestinal tract, and blood. It also helps reduce pain. Greater celandine is also used in the treatment of inflammation of the gallbladder or gallstones. It has antispasmodic properties, which helps to relax the muscles of the various ducts and reduce cramping pains. Take half a teaspoon of the tincture three times per day to benefit from greater celandine's liver-cleansing properties.

Balmony (*Chelone glabra*)

If you are suffering from jaundice or gallbladder problems, you will find balmony helpful. The herb's main use is for gallbladder problems, including inflammation of the gallbladder, due to either infection or gravel or stones. It is particularly good when the gallstones are sufficiently large that they are blocking the flow of bile. If that happens the bile backs up into the liver and is dispersed throughout the bloodstream, causing the yellowing of the skin seen in jaundice. For this purpose, it combines well with goldenseal.

It reduces nausea and vomiting and has stimulant properties. Balmony stimulates the appetite and flow of digestive juices. It is helpful for dyspepsia or heartburn, nausea, and colic. It is also used in expelling worms. Steep two teaspoons of the dried herb per cup of boiled water for ten to fifteen minutes. Drink three cups daily. Alternatively, take one-quarter teaspoon of the tincture three times per day.

Barberry (*Berberis vulgaris*)

The bark, roots, stems, and berries of barberry offer cleansing properties that help with detoxifying the liver and gallbladder. It stimulates the flow of bile and digestive juices, reduces nausea and vomiting, tones and strengthens the body, and stimulates bowel action. It is used for gallbladder problems such as nausea and biliousness, inflammation, and gallstones. It is also helpful for mild to severe liver problems, even those severe enough to cause jaundice. It is effective against microorganisms, including malaria and the fungus *Candida albicans*. Use one teaspoonful of the dried root per cup of boiling water. Drink one cup three times per day. Alternatively, take ¼ to ½ teaspoon of the tincture two to three times per day.

Black Root *(Leptandra virginica)*

The Seneca natives shared their knowledge of black root to help Europeans who came to North America. It stimulates bile flow, promotes perspiration and cleansing through the skin, has antispasmodic properties, and strongly encourages bowel elimination. It is useful in the treatment of cholecystitis or inflamed gallbladder and for liver congestion that may lead to jaundice. It works well with barberry and dandelion for liver congestion. Avoid using the fresh root since it can cause violent vomiting and purging of the bowels. Use black root with care. Use one teaspoon of the dried root per cup of water. Simmer for ten minutes. Drink one cup three times per day. Alternatively, use a quarter to a half teaspoon of the tincture, three times per day.

Blue Flag *(Iris versicolor)*

Blue flag stimulates bile flow and purging of the intestines, reduces inflammation, and cleanses the blood and urinary tract. It is good for eczema and psoriasis, acne, and other skin eruptions. For skin problems, blue flag works well with burdock and yellow dock. Use half to one teaspoon of the dried herb per cup of boiling water. Drink one cup three times daily. Alternatively, use a quarter to a half teaspoon of the tincture three times daily.

Boldo *(Peumus boldo)*

The leaves of this South American herb stimulate bile flow and tone the liver and increase urination to cleanse the urinary tract. Boldo helps with gallbladder inflammation and gallstones, as well as cystitis and fluid retention. It also has sedative properties to help a person relax. Use one teaspoon of the dried leaves per cup of boiling water. Drink one cup three times per day. Alternatively, take one-quarter teaspoon of the tincture three times per day.

Fringetree Bark (*Chionanthus virginicus*)
This powerful liver- and gallbladder-cleansing herb is useful in even severe circumstances. It is helpful for gallstones, gallbladder inflammation, and jaundice. It also normalizes bowel movements. It stimulates bile flow, tones the liver, cleanses blood, and encourages urine flow to cleanse the urinary tract. Make an infusion from one to two teaspoons of the dried herb per cup of boiling water. Let brew for 10 minutes. Drink three cups daily. Alternatively, take one-quarter teaspoon of tincture three times per day.

Vervain (*Verbena officinalis*)
Vervain tones the liver and helps to stimulate normal functioning of both the liver and gallbladder. It is not a primary liver or gallbladder herb but still works well, especially in conjunction with other herbs.

Vervain has antispasmodic properties, calms the nervous system, tones and strengthens the overall body, promotes perspiration and cleansing through the skin, and stimulates breast milk production in women who are nursing infants. Vervain also helps with depression, especially in combination with the herbs skullcap, oats, and lady's slipper. Use between one and three teaspoons of dried herb per cup of water to make an infusion. Drink one cup, three times per day. Alternatively, take a half to one teaspoon of the tincture three times per day.

Wahoo (*Euonymus atropurpureus*)
The bark of this herb is far more useful than its name might suggest. It stimulates the liver, primarily by stimulating bile flow. It is one of the best

liver-cleansing herbs, alongside milk thistle and dandelion. It is good for treating virtually any type of liver and gallbladder problem, including jaundice, gallstones, gallbladder inflammation, and pain. It also cleanses the blood, urinary tract, and intestines. In the latter case, it does so through its laxative effect. Wahoo is also good if you feel sluggish. Make a decoction using a half to one teaspoon of dried herb per cup of water. Drink one cup of this strained mixture, three times per day. Alternatively, you can take a half to one teaspoon of the tincture three times per day.

Yarrow (*Achillea millefolium*)

You learned about yarrow's potent healing abilities for the urinary tract. It is also a good liver cleanser. Two animal studies proved its ability to protect the liver from toxic chemical damage. A study from researchers in India proves its abilities for healing hepatitis.[26] Use one teaspoon of the dried herb (any combination of leaves, flowers, or stems) per cup of boiling water. Drink one cup three times per day.

Astragalus (*Astragalus, various species*)

In addition to cleansing the lymphatic system, astragalus is an excellent liver protector. In his book *The New Healing Herbs*, Michael Castleman cites a study conducted in China, in which mice were given stilbenemide, a cancer chemotherapy drug that causes liver damage. Some mice were given astragalus as well. The ones that received only the drug developed serious liver damage, while those that also took astragalus did not. Astragalus is primarily available as a tincture or in capsule or tablet form. Since potency can vary greatly with this herb, it is best to follow the package directions for the optimum dose.

Supercharge Your Liver and Gallbladder Cleansing

You can employ some powerful energy medicine techniques to improve the cleansing ability of the liver and gallbladder. Two of the best ones include acupressure for these detox organs, and massaging the neurolymphatic massage points that are linked to the gall-bladder and liver.

Acupressure for Liver Cleansing
+ Heart 8 (H 8) is located on the palm of the hand, about one inch below the webbing between the little finger and ring finger.
+ Liver 2 (Liv 2) is located on the top of the foot where the big toe and the second toe meet.

Then:
+ Lung 8 (Lu 8) is located on the inside of the arm, on the thumb side, about one inch higher than the wrist crease.
+ Liver 4 (Liv 4) is located on the front of the ankle bone on the inside of the leg.

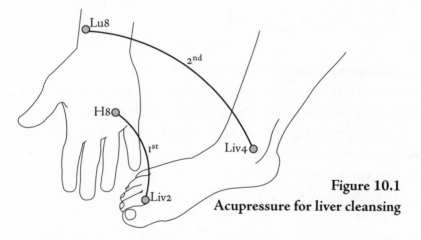

Figure 10.1
Acupressure for liver cleansing

Acupressure for Gallbladder Cleansing
+ Small Intestine 5 (SI 5) is located on the back of the hand at the level of the wrist, on the little finger side.
+ Gallbladder 38 (GB 38) is located on the outside of the lower leg, several inches above the ankle in a depression where the two bones meet.

Then:

- Large Intestine 1 (LI 1) is located on the outside edge (the thumb side) of the index finger at the base of the nail.
- Gallbladder 44 (GB 44) is located on the outside edge of the fourth toe (nearest the little toe) at the base of the toenail.

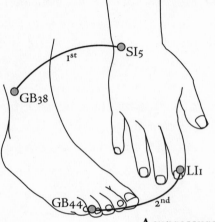

Figure 10.2
Acupressure for gallbladder cleansing

Massage to Enhance Liver and Gallbladder Cleansing

You can massage parts of the lymphatic system that correspond with the liver and gallbladder. These include the following:

- under the right breast, from the outside edge of the ribs to the middle of the body;
- under the inside edge of the third and fourth ribs; and
- about an inch on either side of the spine between the shoulder blades.

Vigorously massage the areas mentioned above, which you will find in the following diagram (Fig. 10.3). These areas are much larger than acupressure points, so don't worry if you're on the right spot. If it feels tender to rub, you've found the right spots. You can be fully clothed while spending a minute or two vigorously massaging these areas.

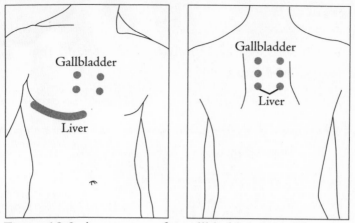

Figure 10.3 Acupressure for gallbladder cleansing

Cleansing your liver and gallbladder on a regular basis gives these two valuable organs the boost they need to perform over five hundred functions. Consider your detoxification efforts for these organs comparable to insurance. By restoring the health of the liver and gallbladder through periodic cleansing, you are helping to ensure the health of hundreds of processes in your body, all of which are essential to great health.

In this chapter you learned
  + The gallbladder and liver perform over 500 important functions
  + There are many symptoms and disorders linked with an unhealthy liver and gallbladder
  + It is critical to great health that you cleanse your liver and gallbladder
  + Particular foods, herbs, and energy medicine techniques assist with liver and gallbladder detoxification

References

1. Frances Albrecht, "The Basics of Detoxing Your Liver," *Healthwell*, April 1997.

2. Scott Rigden, "Liver Detoxification," www.drscottrigden.com.

3. Sandra Cabot, *The Liver Cleansing Diet* (Scottsdale, AZ: SCB International, Inc., 2000).

4. Cabot, *The Liver Cleansing Diet*.

5. "Fat-Burning Foods," *Woman's World*, April 27, 2004.

6. "Fat-Burning Foods."

7. "Fat-Burning Foods."

8. "Fat-Burning Foods."

9. "Fat-Burning Foods."

10. "Fat-Burning Foods."

11. "Fat-Burning Foods."

12. "Fat-Burning Foods."

13. Ann Louise Gittleman, *The Fat Flush Plan* (New York, NY: McGraw-Hill, 2002), p. 35.

14. Gittleman, *The Fat Flush Plan*, p. 19.

15. Gittleman, *The Fat Flush Plan*, p. 35.

16. Gittleman, *The Fat Flush Plan*, p. 42.

17. Albrecht, "The Basics of Detoxing Your Liver."

18. Cabot, *The Liver Cleansing Diet*, p. 69.

19. "Are You Taking the Life Out of Your Liver?" www.greatamericanproducts.com.

20. Xandria Williams, *The Herbal Detox Plan* (Carlsbad, CA: Hay House, Inc., 2003), p. 129.

21. Gittleman, *The Fat Flush Plan*, p. 20.

22. Gittleman, *The Fat Flush Plan*, p. 20.

23. Cabot, *The Liver Cleansing Diet*, p. 68.

24. Gittleman, *The Fat Flush Plan*, pp. 19–20.

25. Albrecht, "The Basics of Detoxing Your Liver."

26. Michael Castleman, *The New Healing Herbs* (New York, NY: Bantam Books, 2001), p. 607.

CHAPTER 11

Targeting the Blood, Lungs, and Skin

"Live each season as it passes; breathe the air, drink the drink, taste the fruit, and resign yourself to the influences of each."

Henry David Thoreau

In this chapter you will learn

* The many important functions of the blood, lungs, and skin
* The symptoms and disorders linked with excessive toxins in the blood, lungs, or absorbed by the skin
* Why it is essential to purify your blood and cleanse the lungs and skin of toxins
* How to use foods, herbs, breathing exercises, massage and energy medicine to assist with cleansing your blood, lungs, and skin

Maintaining healthy blood, lungs, and skin is essential to great health. Your blood bathes the cells of your body and provides them oxygen that is essential to life. Your lungs and respiratory system ensure that your blood has this oxygen available—every cell depends on their optimal functioning. Your skin plays an integral protective and cleansing role for your body. What the other detox systems cannot handle, your skin tries to eliminate. If you are suffering from skin problems, look no further than inadequate detoxification mechanisms for the solution.

During Phase 4 of *The 4-Week Ultimate Body Detox Plan* we targeted the blood and circulatory systems, lungs and respiratory tract, and the skin. To modify, extend, or deepen the 4-week cleanse, you can use additional herbal therapy, nutritional therapy, and other types of natural treatments, including herbal teas, green food supplement, and Cellfood®. You can incorporate these suggestions into the four-week plan for power-packed cleansing or you can further cleanse these systems after the four weeks are completed. The program described in Chapter 5 is recommended, along with the suggested therapies below.

I have included information about many excellent herbs for cleansing the blood, lungs, and skin at the end of each respective section. Herbs are powerful medicine, so consult a medical doctor before using any herbs if you are pregnant or have a serious health condition. Consult an herbalist before combining two or more herbs or while taking medication with herbs. Avoid long-term use of any herb (longer than three weeks) without first consulting a qualified herbalist.

BLOOD AND CIRCULATORY SYSTEM

Sixty thousand miles of veins and arteries, along with your heart, pump approximately five litres of blood, oxygen, and nutrients throughout your body every minute. Along with all this blood, your circulatory system is often loaded with plaque and cholesterol buildup, thanks to our love of french fries, ice cream, burgers, cakes, and all things artery-clogging. Sugar and sweets and everything grease, that is what heart disease is made of. If you think you are safe, you may wish to consider that one in every two people will die of heart disease or stroke. That's right, over 50 percent of people living in the Western world die of diseases that have an underlying cause of hardening of the arteries (also called atherosclerosis or arteriosclerosis).[1] That need not happen if we keep our arteries cleaner.

You may have heard the words "plaque," "LDL," and "HDL" cholesterol floating around. LDL is also commonly called the "bad" cholesterol while HDL is sometimes called the "good" cholesterol. You have probably been exposed to people talking about triglycerides and homocysteine, as well. These are not the stuff of a chemistry experiment, unless you are referring to the myriad chemical reactions taking place within your body. To help end the confusion of all this medical jargon: plaque is the buildup that occurs in your arteries, never your veins. Arteries have an inner muscular layer that veins lack. This muscle wall constricts and expands, increasing blood pressure, whereas veins have a lower pressure.

Plaque is not just one thing; it is made up of many substances, including fibrin, collagen, phospholipids, triglycerides, cholesterol, mucopolysaccharides, foreign proteins, heavy metals, muscle tissue, and debris—bonded together with calcium.[2] It is not necessary to know about all these substances—suffice it to say that cholesterol is getting a negative reputation and being wrongfully blamed as the sole cause of heart disease. Your body needs cholesterol to live. According to some experts, cholesterol prevents blood cells from being damaged by the acidity and free radicals in the bloodstream. Cholesterol may be a potent antioxidant that protects your body against free radicals.

All the unhealthy foods I mentioned above create acidity in the body. This acidity scours the walls of the arteries, according to some experts. Cholesterol, which is primarily made in your body, attempts to protect the arteries by patching their inner walls. High cholesterol is not a disease. According to Dr. David Rowland, author of *The Nutritional Bypass*, "It is a symptom of insults to our bodies through lack of exercise and improper diet." One of the most common questions I am asked is whether high cholesterol levels can be normalized using food. I tell people, "Food is one of the main factors for high cholesterol levels—the wrong food, that is. Eating the right foods and exercising can reverse it."

There are numerous ways to get and keep your blood and circulatory system working more efficiently. Of course, there are the obvious ways: stop eating so much meat, dairy products, sugar and sweets, fried and prepared foods. Stop adding salt to your foods. In a week or so, your taste buds will adapt and you will actually enjoy the taste of foods better. Most people know these nutritional basics and simply make poor choices, perhaps believing that they are indestructible, or maybe they just do not care enough. Some people believe that only food that is bad for you actually tastes good. This could not be farther from the truth. The best-tasting food I have ever eaten is healthy. Chapter 13 contains many excellent recipes to help you discover the decadent taste of healthy foods.

You learned earlier that the kidneys filter the blood, so it is imperative to cleanse the kidneys when dealing with any cardio-vascular problems.

Blood and Circulatory System Stress Quiz

Do your fingers and/or toes frequently go cold?

Do you suffer from chest pains after physical exertion or emotional stress?

Have you been diagnosed with high blood pressure?

Do your arms and/or legs often "fall asleep"?

Do you have a sharp, diagonal crease in your earlobe?

Does a short walk cause cramping or pain in your legs?

Do you become breathless with even a slight exertion or from lying down?

Do you urinate more than twice during the night?

Do you have a persistent cough?

Is your memory not as good as it used to be?

Do you get tingling in your lips or fingers?

Do your hands cramp from writing?

Do your ankles swell in the evening?

If you answered yes to any of these questions, your heart and circulatory system could use further tuning up.

Eat for Clean Blood and Circulatory System

The topic of arterial cleansing is a book unto itself. Some forms of nutritional chelation can speed the cleansing of the arteries. Nutritional chelation is a method of taking large amounts of specific nutrients that are proven to break down plaque and escort it out of the body.[3] The topic is too voluminous for adequate discussion here. See the Resources section for information on nutritional chelation.

In addition to eating a nutritious diet of wholesome foods, primarily or exclusively vegetarian, with large amounts of fruits, vegetables, and whole grains and legumes, you can also supplement with particular nutrients and herbs that are beneficial in helping to break down plaque buildup.

Boosting your levels of HDL cholesterol will help lessen the amount of LDL cholesterol and triglyceride levels, two of the key constituents of plaque. You can increase the levels of your body's natural vacuum cleaner by adding a greater number of flavonoids to your diet. The best sources are fruits and vegetables, especially pitted fruits such as apricots, peaches, plums, and cherries. Niacin (vitamin B3) is also important to increase this good cholesterol.

Eating a diet high in fibre is essential to flush the arteries. Choose carefully, however, since all fibres are not created equal. Water-insoluble fibres such as wheat bran and cellulose, are minimally effective in lowering the risk of arteriosclerosis. Water-soluble fibre such as that found in oats, psyllium, guar gum, and pectin are far more effective.[4]

Folate (vitamin B9) is important to lower excess homocysteine that could be prematurely damaging and aging your body's cells, which will speed up the aging process. Oranges are rich in folate.

Getting adequate amounts of essential fatty acids is also imperative to flush out toxins and plaque buildup in the arteries. We discussed the different types of essential fatty acids earlier. Most people eat a ratio of about 20:1 of omega-6 fatty acids to omega-3 fatty acids. The ideal ratio, estimated by experts, is 1:2 in favour of larger amounts of omega-3 fatty acids. This means that most people are eating twenty times more omega-6 fatty acids than they should be. Omega-3s play an integral role in cleansing the arteries and preventing heart disease and stroke. Some of the best sources of omega-3s are raw unsalted walnuts, flax seeds, and cold-pressed flax seed oil. All these ingredients should be found in the refrigerator section of a health food or grocery store, otherwise their critical ingredients might be rancid by the time you get them. They should also be kept in the refrigerator at home. Grind flax seeds in a small coffee grinder prior to adding them to salads, salad dressings, or smoothies or sprinkling them on whole-grain cereal or toast. Do not cook any of these ingredients, otherwise you will turn them from healthy fatty acids to damaging trans fats.

Clean Up Your Blood and Circulatory System

If you have not already quit smoking and you answered yes to any of the above questions, it is time to quit now. Smoking is directly linked with circulatory disorders and heart disease. Truthfully, it is a slow suicide. Instead of pulling a trigger on a gun or using some other violent means to die, a person slowly poisons every cell in his or her body. Smokers die many years earlier than non-smokers. They typically die of heart disease or cancer.

Adequate exercise is essential to cleansing the arteries. When you undertake aerobic activities such as walking, jogging, Pilates, and other vigorous activities, your heart rate increases, thereby quickening the pace of blood that pumps through your arteries. This is critical to adequately cleanse the arteries. Exercise also helps lower your levels of HDL cholesterol, which in turn lessens LDL cholesterol and triglycerides. Research shows that cardiovascular exercise for thirty minutes at a time, three times per week, has a significant effect on high cholesterol levels.[5]

Herbs for Deep Blood and Circulatory System Cleansing

Aloe Vera

Aloe vera juice is helpful for cleansing your arteries. Aloe vera is a tropical plant that has been used medicinally for millennia. Its healing properties have been known for over four thousand years. It has been used for stomach and intestinal ailments, dysentery and kidney infections, and sunburns, and to slow the aging process, but it is also effective against arterial plaque. Aloe vera encourages circulation and elimination. It is full of amino acids, enzymes, chlorophyll, essential oils, vitamins and minerals, and other nutrients that are beneficial for good health.

Herbalists know aloe vera for its antibacterial, antiviral, painkilling, anti-inflammatory, fever-reducing, and cleansing properties. It also helps dilate capillaries and enhances normal cell growth, making it useful for treating diseases such as arteriosclerosis and cancer.

Drink a quarter to half a cup of aloe vera juice, twice a day. Note that aloe vera juice is not the same as the gel, which tends to be more concentrated. Avoid using "aloes" or "aloe latex" since their strong purgative action can be too harsh on the intestinal tract and result in severe cramping or diarrhea. Avoid aloe vera juice during pregnancy and lactation.

Yellow Dock *(Rumex crispus)*

Yellow dock is an excellent blood-cleansing herb that also benefits the skin, intestines, and mildly stimulates the liver. It has antiviral properties as well. Use one to two teaspoons of dried herb per cup of water to make a decoction. Drink one cup three times per day. Alternatively, take a quarter to a half teaspoon of the tincture three times per day.

LUNGS AND RESPIRATORY TRACT

The respiratory tract has numerous parts, including the nose, pharynx, hypopharynx, larynx, vocal cords, trachea, and lungs. Air enters the trachea, where it moves into passageways called bronchi or bronchial tubes that are located behind the rib cage. From there it moves into smaller tubes called bronchioles and then into even smaller air sacs called alveolar sacs or alveoli, where oxygen is extracted and supplied to millions of capillaries. At that point, oxygen combines with hemoglobin in red blood cells and is carried throughout the body. Exhaling reverses the passage from alveoli to the trachea to allow carbon dioxide to be released.

Asthma, bronchitis, and emphysema are breathing disorders linked to improper lung functioning or damage to the lungs. Any of these disorders, or other lung problems, can be triggered or worsened by toxins, particularly those found in the air, such as cigarette smoke. The lungs have the greatest exposure of all the internal organs to the outside world. Air includes dust and pollution, chemicals and microorganisms, all of which enter the lungs and need to be separated from oxygen.

Enzymes naturally found in the lungs help metabolize chemicals such as medications. These enzymes break down synthetic chemicals to make them more water-soluble so they can be excreted by the kidneys.

If you are suffering from lung or respiratory tract problems or disorders, you can do a great deal to ease your difficulties. After completing *The 4-Week Ultimate Body Detox Plan*, you may wish to further target the lungs.

Lung and Respiratory System Stress Quiz

Do you suffer from a chronic cough?
Do you frequently have a runny nose?
Do you have frequent bouts of bronchitis or wheezing?
Do you have frequent or ongoing sinus problems?
Do you suffer from asthma or other breathing disorders?
Do you suffer from allergies?

If you answered yes to any of these questions, your lungs and respiratory system could use further tuning up.

Eat for Clean Lungs and Respiratory System

Supplement with vitamin E. This antioxidant helps protect the lungs from toxins and their resulting damage.

Drink at least eight to twelve glasses of water, unsweetened juice, herb teas, and soup broth per day.

Avoid all dairy products. Many people are sensitive to these foods without realizing that their sensitivity is showing up in chronic health problems. Even if you are *not* sensitive to dairy, these foods are quite mucus-forming. They add further burden to the lungs and respiratory tract. Yes, I know, "but, where will you get your calcium?" The answer to this is simple and we've already discussed it briefly. You will get your calcium from the same sources as every other animal (we are part of the animal kingdom, after all) on the planet. Most foods contain calcium. Don't forget what I explained earlier: just because there is plenty of calcium in dairy products does not mean that you should eat them, nor does it mean that your body will extract the calcium from this food. Eliminate them from your diet and, over time, your lungs will thank you. Contrary to popular belief, so will your bones (for more information, consult my book, *Healing Injuries the Natural Way (www.healinginjuries.com)*).

Eat plenty of fruits and vegetables and gluten-free grains such as millet and brown rice. You can learn how to prepare these grains in Chapter 13. Gluten sensitivities often mask themselves as lung and respiratory conditions.

Eat chlorophyll-rich foods. Chlorophyll is the green colour in most plant foods. Eat lots of leafy greens and supplement your diet with "green supplements" such as chlorella, spirulina, or barley green, all of which enhance lung cleansing.

Eat one to two tablespoons of ground flax seeds daily, sprinkled on food after it has been cooked (do not heat or cook flax seeds) or mixed into smoothies. Flax seeds are helpful in soothing and protecting lung tissue while helping to alleviate coughs and helping the lungs ward off infection.

Eat apples, blueberries, bilberries, onions, green tea, and fruits that contain pits, which include apricots, peaches, plums, and cherries. They are high in natural substances called flavonoids. These substances are powerful antioxidants that reduce the damage of toxins in your body. They also bind to heavy metals. Plants produce these substances to protect themselves from bacteria, parasites, and cellular damage. More than four thousand of these powerful substances are currently known. Some flavonoids found in fruits and veggies contain more powerful antioxidants than vitamins C, E, or beta-carotene. Flavonoids even protect these vitamins from damage so they can work their magic in your body. So there are four thousand more reasons to eat your fruits and vegetables.

Clean Up Your Lungs and Respiratory System

I hope it is not necessary to tell you that if you are suffering from any lung or respiratory tract disorders or ailments, you should avoid all forms of cigarette smoke. That includes second-hand smoke, which many studies have shown is actually more harmful than smoking.

If you have not already stopped using scented and synthetic cleaning products, personal hygiene products, cosmetics, body- and hair-care products, it is essential that you do so now if you want to give your lungs a chance to recover.

Try to minimize your exposure to dust, dust mites, mould, and pollens if you suspect you are allergic. I have seen many allergic clients who gave up dairy products and refined sugars recover from their seasonal allergies. If you have allergies you might benefit from taking quail egg homogenate. Quail breeders accidentally led doctors, especially French researcher J.C. Truffier, to study the effects of quail eggs as an allergy remedy. A French woman who was a new quail breeder and allergy and asthma sufferer saw her allergies and asthma disappear as she ate more quail eggs. This observation led Dr. Truffier, followed by over two hundred allergists, to prescribe six raw quail eggs per day as a treatment for allergies, with tremendous success. However, eating six raw quail eggs per day has obvious problems. Scientists in France later developed a tablet that dissolves under the tongue while delivering the anti-allergy benefits of eating the eggs. Many clinical trials have proven quail eggs effective for the treatment of allergic asthma, sinusitis, and hay fever symptoms. See the Resources at the back of this book if you are unable to find quail egg homogenate.

Improving the air quality in your home (and workplace, if possible) should be a priority if you suffer from respiratory ailments. In addition to improving the quality of cleaning products and building materials, using a high-quality air purifier can help.

Exercise is imperative to help clear the lungs of excess mucus and toxins. The increased oxygen helps the lungs perform their jobs more efficiently while helping you to feel more energized due to the increased oxygen available throughout your body's cells for cleansing and healing. Be careful not to over-exercise if you have breathing difficulties as this can worsen problems. Gradually build your tolerance for cardiovascular activities.

Breathing and emotional releasing exercises like those suggested in Chapters 6 and 7 will also be helpful to oxygenate your body and improve the functioning of the respiratory tract. They take minimal time and effort yet offer tremendous rewards. Even someone who is very ill with respiratory problems can typically handle qigong breathing exercises like those you learned earlier in this book.

Herbs for Deep Lung and Respiratory System Cleaning

Coltsfoot (*Tussilago farfara*)

Coltsfoot is an excellent herb for clearing out excess mucus from the lungs and bronchial tubes. In addition to clearing catarrh, it helps soothe coughs, protects and soothes mucous membranes, and increases the flow of urine to help with urinary tract toxins. It has proven itself useful for bronchitis, chronic and acute coughs, asthma, whooping cough, and emphysema. It combines well with horehound and comfrey. You can use one to two teaspoons of dried herb per cup for an infusion or use a half to one teaspoon three times a day in tincture form.

Comfrey (*Symphytum officinale*)

Comfrey soothes and protects the body's mucous membranes while helping to clear out excess phlegm and mucus. It also soothes irritable coughs and bronchitis. It combines well with borage. Comfrey works on damaged mucous membranes in the digestive tract and is therefore helpful for hiatus hernia, stomach or duodenal ulcers, inflammation of the small or large intestines, ulcerative colitis (especially combined with slippery elm powder and aloe vera juice), and skin problems. Use one to three teaspoons of finely chopped herb per cup of water for an infusion or use a half to one teaspoon of tincture three times a day.

Daisy (*Bellis perennis*)

Use the flower heads, not the leaves, dried or fresh. If you are using fresh, be sure that it is the correct species and that the plant is organic. Daisy is an expectorant that helps to clear out excess mucus from the lungs while toning the tissues. It combines well with coltsfoot or goldenrod. It also helps if you are cleansing too quickly and have diarrhea. Daisy is also helpful for rheumatism, arthritis, liver, and kidney problems. Use one teaspoon of the dried flower heads per cup of water for an infusion, drinking one cup three to four times a day. Alternatively, use a half to one teaspoon of the tincture, three times a day.

Elecampane (*Inula helenium*)

The root of the elecampane plant helps kill harmful bacteria, lessens coughs, expels excess mucus, and helps alleviate stomach problems. In the respiratory system, it gradually alleviates any fever that might be present while battling infection and maximizing excretion of toxins through perspiration. If you have a tickling cough or bronchitis, elecampane may be able to help. Because of its action on excess mucus and toxins in the respiratory tract, it is often helpful with emphysema, asthma, bronchial asthma, and tuberculosis. In addition to the effects on the respiratory tract, it also helps a sluggish digestive system. Take one teaspoon of herb per cup of water in an infusion or one to two millilitres of tincture, three times a day.

Grindelia (*Grindelia camporum*)
If you have problems with catarrh, grindelia is the herb of choice. It is especially helpful for eliminating excess catarrh from the upper respiratory tract while helping to relax the muscles of the lungs and bronchial tubes, making it suitable for people suffering from asthma and bronchial disorders or whooping cough. It is also appropriate for lung disorders that are accompanied by an increase in heartbeat or nervous tension. In addition, it helps normalize high blood pressure since it helps relax the smooth muscles of the heart and arteries through its antispasmodic action. This herb combines well with lobelia and pillbearing spurge. Take one teaspoon of the dried herb in a cup of water and infuse for ten to fifteen minutes. Drink this amount three times a day. Alternatively, take a quarter to a half teaspoon of tincture three times a day.

Horehound (*Marrubium vulgare*)
While you may prefer the candy from this bitter herb, it is the dried leaves that are best for their medicinal properties. They relax the muscles of the lungs while encouraging the clearing of excess mucus. Due to its antispasmodic properties, it is also good for bronchial spasms and coughs. Thanks to its highly bitter nature (which is why it is frequently blended with sugar) it is also good for digestive difficulties. The same bitter nature stimulates bile flow, thereby helping to cleanse the digestive tract by initiating normal elimination from the intestines. Horehound combines well with coltsfoot, mullein, and lobelia to effectively clear the lungs. Take one teaspoon of dried herb per cup of water or a quarter to a half teaspoon of tincture three times a day.

Lobelia (*Lobelia inflata*)

Lobelia is an excellent herb for lung concerns, coughs, infections, bronchial asthma, and excessive phlegm. It helps alleviate bronchial spasms, making it useful for asthmatics. It is an extremely strong herb and should therefore be used with caution. Infuse a quarter to a half teaspoon of dried herb per cup and drink one cup three times a day. Alternatively, take one-eighth to one-quarter teaspoon of tincture three times a day.

Lungwort (*Pulmonaria officinalis*)

Lungwort clears catarrh from the upper respiratory tract, nose, throat, and upper bronchial tubes, while helping the body soothe the mucous membranes in these regions and lessening coughs. It is also good for bronchitis. Lungwort combines well with coltsfoot, lobelia, and horehound. As an infusion, mix one to two teaspoons of dried herb per cup and drink one cup three times a day. Alternatively, take a quarter to one teaspoon of tincture three times a day.

Mullein (*Verbascum thapsus*)

The leaves and flowers of the mullein plant soothe mucous membranes in the respiratory tract while clearing excess mucus. It reduces inflammation and pain, including within the nasal lining, throat, bronchial tubes, and digestive tract. Mullein is also mildly cleansing for the urinary tract. It is helpful for coughs, sore throats, and bronchitis. Use one to two teaspoons of dried herb per cup of water to make infusions. Drink one cup three times a day. Alternatively, take a quarter to one teaspoon of tincture three times a day.

Pleurisy Root (*Aescepias tuberosa*)

Pleurisy root is another good herb for clearing out excess catarrh and mucus from the respiratory tract. It also has antispasmodic properties, decreases flatulence, and increases urine flow to help expel toxins within the urinary tract. If you are suffering from a large amount of mucous or catarrhal buildup, pleurisy root works better when combined with coltsfoot. If you are suffering from chronic respiratory problems, including asthma, combine pleurisy root with lobelia. To make an infusion, combine a half to one teaspoon of dried herb per cup of water. Drink one cup three times a day. You can substitute a quarter to a half teaspoon of tincture three times a day if you prefer.

Red Clover (*Trifolium pratense*)

You are probably far more familiar with red clover than you realize. It rears its head in lawns across the country, and most people respond by pulling out their nasty chemical weed killers. What you may not realize that this so-called weed is one of Nature's powerful medicines. Red clover helps to expel excess mucus from the respiratory tract and is an excellent blood purifier. Use one to three teaspoons of dried red clover flowers per cup of boiling water. Let infuse for ten to fifteen minutes. Drink one cup of this infusion three times a day. Alternatively, use one teaspoon of red clover tincture three times daily.

Pokeroot (*Phytolacca americana*)

Pokeroot, as you learned earlier, is an excellent choice for cleansing the lymphatic system. Pokeroot is also helpful in expelling excess catarrh and dealing with general respiratory conditions. It is also a powerful blood cleanser. Take three to ten drops of the tincture in water (warm or cold) daily. Avoid exceeding the recommended dose of this herb.

Supercharge Your Lung Cleansing Efforts

You can massage along the midpoint where the ribs in the front of your body converge, called the sternum, to assist with lung and skin cleansing, according to Donna Eden and David Feinstein. They recommend massaging the sternum, and in the points beneath each of the second, third, and fourth ribs. In addition, massage the points about an inch away from either side of the spine near the top of the shoulder blades. See the diagram below for help finding these spots on the body. These are neurolymphatic massage points that are integrally linked to the lungs. By stimulating them through vigorous massage for a minute or two daily, you will greatly assist with the cleansing efforts of the lungs and skin.

THE SKIN YOU LIVE IN

The skin is the largest organ in your body. Not only does it provide a barrier between your body and the external environment in which you live, it also helps the other detoxification systems cleanse your body of internal toxins. Much of what you slather on your skin will be absorbed. That is why it is imperative that you refrain from using soaps, creams, and other hygiene or beauty products that contain synthetic ingredients. Not only will using them expose you to further toxins, it will also limit your skin's ability to eliminate internal toxins.

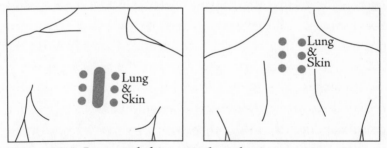

Figure 11.1 Lung and skin neurolymphatic massage points

The skin is mostly waterproof and prevents your body from becoming waterlogged or from drying out. It also protects your body from microorganisms, sun damage, and exposure to cold or heat. Sweat glands lie within the inner part of the skin and produce sweat to prevent the body from overheating. Toxins are also eliminated through sweat.

Skin Stress Quiz

Do you suffer from acne, blackheads, or whiteheads?

Do you ever have rashes or hives?

Do you have psoriasis, eczema, or dry, scaly patches of skin?

Do you have blotchy or ruddy skin?

Do you suffer from dry and/or flaky skin?

If you answered yes to any of these questions, your skin could use cleansing.

Eat for Better Skin

Follow the nutritional suggestions in Chapter 5. If you are still suffering from skin conditions, follow the nutritional and herbal suggestions made under all the other detoxification organs. Often, skin conditions are the result of the other organs being overloaded with toxins.

Herbs for Deep Skin Cleansing

People spend so much money on skin-care and beauty products to improve their skin. Yet what you do internally is far more effective. Let's use our car analogy again. This is like spray-painting a rusting car that is falling apart. It will look slightly improved but the rust will start to show through and the car will still be falling apart.

The skin is a type of run-off system for the other detoxification organs. If you are having skin problems, it could be a sign of a sluggish liver, intestines, blood, or lymphatic system. Work on cleansing the other systems first. Some herbs are specifically good for improving skin problems. Interestingly, they typically cleanse other detox systems at the same time, which could explain their effectiveness.

Yellow Dock (*Rumex crispus*)

Yellow dock is helpful for skin conditions such as acne and psoriasis. It works especially well on the skin when combined with burdock and pokeroot. It is a mild liver stimulant and is sometimes used to treat jaundice. Yellow dock also cleanses the blood, has antiviral properties, and has a mild laxative effect on the intestines. Use one to two teaspoons of dried herb per cup of water to make a decoction. Drink one cup three times a day. Alternatively, take a quarter to a half teaspoon of the tincture three times a day.

Cleavers *(Galium aperine)*
You learned about this plant for its ability to cleanse the kidneys and lymphatic system. Used regularly, it also cleanses the skin and helps with acne. It is best used as an infusion. For cleavers (also known as **Goosegrass** or **Grip Grass**) tea, use two to three teaspoons of the dried herb per cup of water. Drink one cup three times daily. Alternatively, use a half to one teaspoon of tincture three times per day. Avoid using cleavers if you suffer with diabetes or have diabetic tendencies.

Supercharge Your Skin Cleansing Efforts
Follow the directions listed under "Supercharge Your Lung Cleansing Efforts" above. This energy medicine technique is helpful for cleansing both the lungs and skin.

Cleansing your blood and circulatory system, lungs and respiratory system, and skin is essential to health. Keep these powerful detox organs functioning at their best and you will be blessed with more energy, vitality, and freedom from illness.

In this chapter you learned
+ The blood, lungs, and skin play critical roles in great health
+ There are many symptoms and disorders linked with excessive toxins in the blood, lungs, or absorbed by the skin
+ It is essential to purify your blood and cleanse the lungs and skin of toxins to achieve great health
+ Foods, herbs, breathing exercises, massage and energy medicine assist with cleansing your blood, lungs, and skin

References

1. David W. Rowland, *The Nutritional Bypass* (Parry Sound, ON: Rowland Publications, 1999), p. 10.

2. Rowland, *The Nutritional Bypass*, p. 10.

3. Rowland, *The Nutritional Bypass*, p. 6.

4. Rowland, *The Nutritional Bypass*, p. 50.

5. Rowland, *The Nutritional Bypass*, p. 21.

CHAPTER 12

Complementary Detox Therapies

"Healing...is not a science,
but the intuitive art of wooing Nature."
W. H. Auden

In this chapter you will learn
+ Many powerful natural therapies support detoxification
+ Incorporating some of the best detoxification therapies into The 4 Week Ultimate Body Detox Plan will assist your cleansing efforts
+ Some of the best natural therapies for assisting with detoxification include: acupuncture, Alexander technique, aromatherapy, Bach flower remedies, Bowen technique, cranio-sacral therapy, energy medicine or energy kinesiology, far-infrared sauna therapy, homeopathy, lymphatic drainage, massage, naturopathy and natural medicine, osteopathy, quantum biofeedback, reiki, shiatsu, and Thai massage

There are many powerful therapies that can enhance your body's ability to detoxify. Some of my favourites include acupuncture, Alexander Technique, aromatherapy, Bach flower therapy, Bowen Technique, cranio-sacral, energy medicine or energy kinesiology, far-infrared sauna therapy, homeopathy, lymphatic drainage, massage, naturopathy, osteopathy, quantum biofeedback, Reiki, shiatsu, and Thai yoga massage. I discussed a number of these therapies and techniques in Chapter 7, but I believe it is worth reinforcing those ideas in the pages that follow.

While these therapies are not essential elements of *The 4-Week Ultimate Body Detox Plan*, they are highly recommended treatments that can greatly assist with detoxification. I have provided some basic information about each form of therapy to help you decide which one or ones you would like to add to your program. Of course, personal preference, budget, time availability, and access to the therapies will affect your decision about which therapies to pursue.

The role the therapy plays in helping with detoxification varies greatly from one to another. I have included information about the ways each therapy assists with detox below.

ACUPUNCTURE[1]

Acupuncture is a powerful healing modality that assists your body with detoxification. It is a highly respected form of medicine that is far older than "modern medicine"; acupuncture is at least five thousand years old. By some anthropological findings, it may even be ten thousand years old.

It works on several different premises, but the main one is the energy of the body, which acupuncturists refer to as "chi" or "qi" (both are pronounced "chee"). This energy, or life force, is found in the body, air, water, and food, and while it may be invisible, it is scientifically proven to be integral to life.

In Chinese philosophy, there are two main streams of life force energy, called yin and yang. Balancing these energies in the body is essential to optimum health. Excessive toxins in an organ, joint, fatty deposits, or other cells or tissues can disrupt the natural flow of energy throughout the body, resulting in pain, inflammation, or myriad other symptoms.

There are many different types of acupuncturists. They may use varying methods of diagnosis to determine the right acupuncture points for inserting needles. The most common ones include tongue diagnosis, pulse diagnosis, questioning you about your symptoms and what makes them better or worse, and face reading, which entails collecting visual clues from your face or eyes.

The acupuncturist will select which points he or she will use to bring balance back to the system and then insert fine needles into those areas. Most people barely feel the insertion of these needles, which are much finer than a pin. Acupuncture is renowned for pain relief. In China, most hospitals do not use anaesthesia drugs; instead, they rely on acupuncture anaesthesia for major and minor surgeries and pain relief.

Acupuncture is especially helpful for dealing with toxic buildup in the joints, organs, and tissues that may be disrupting the proper flow of energy in the body. If you have pain, acupuncture can usually help. Most acupuncturists will recommend two or three sessions per week for the first three weeks. Afterward, he or she will determine the frequency of visits based on necessity and severity of your health concerns.

ALEXANDER TECHNIQUE

Frederick Mathias Alexander was an Australian actor at the turn of the nineteenth century. Alexander suffered from chronic voice problems that threatened his acting career, particularly because his problems would usually coincide with his presence on the stage. He began to study his movement and posture in the mirror, mimicking his acting roles for clues. Alexander noticed that he frequently shifted his head in a manner that increased the stress on his neck, throat, and breathing. As a result of certain postural re-alignments and the correction of negative attitudinal patterns, he found that he was able to influence a number of health concerns. The Alexander Technique was born and is now widely practised as an effective therapy for raising awareness of the importance of correct bodily positions while lying, sitting, standing, and walking.

Incorrect posture creates additional stress on the body and stress can contribute to increased states of toxicity. While the Alexander Technique is primarily used to help people with pain and injuries, it can play an important role in making our bodies more efficient, effective, and comfortable. It has been used to successfully treat rounded shoulders, stoops, backaches, tight neck and throat, headaches, carpal tunnel syndrome, arthritis, and even respiratory conditions.

Alexander Technique is non-invasive. The practitioner will gently guide you through different postures and positions that promote health by minimizing the stress on your spine, muscles, nerves, and soft tissue.

AROMATHERAPY

Aromatherapy is as old as nature itself. The scents of flowers, trees, and other plants have always had an impact on other life forms. Archaeological evidence has demonstrated that the ancient civilizations of Egypt, Greece, and Rome were familiar with the use of aromatherapy oils. And while modern exploration of this wonderful form of therapy became more widespread in the last century, the healing properties of these truly natural oils have been confirmed in the laboratories of leading universities and research institutes worldwide. These potent essential oils have produced remarkable results on pain, inflammation, infection, depression, dementia, and many other symptoms.

The great thing about aromatherapy is… everything. Fragrant scented oils are gently applied through massage or inhaled after being diffused into the air. It seems too good to be effective medicine but an experienced aromatherapist can achieve excellent results through the application of the correct essential oil. The science behind aromatherapy involves signals transmitted from cells in the nose to the brain. The message sent to the brain varies with the scent or scents detected by the nose. The brain then transmits signals to the rest of the body, which again acts accordingly.

Aromatherapy oil may consist of a single plant oil or a combination of many different oils from many species. The oils frequently have more than one therapeutic use based on their properties. The three main classifications are "uplifting," "balancing," and "calming." Choosing the appropriate oil also involves choosing high-quality oils. The therapeutic benefits of aromatherapy are greatly diminished if the processing compromises the product (i.e., the integrity of the plant or plants). You are not likely to find quality aromatherapy products in most of the "bath and body" chain stores or department stores, including many popular ones. And remember: the last thing you want in your detoxification program is more chemicals, so avoid oils that are labelled "fragrance" or include ingredients other than oils from the plant or plants they are supposed to comprise. Choose only high-quality oils to avoid toxic, rancid oils that are common in bath and beauty stores.

BACH FLOWER REMEDIES

As we discussed earlier in this book, British medical doctor and bacteriologist Dr. Edward Bach founded a system of treating emotional imbalances using the "essence" of flowers. Bach believed, as many other health practitioners do, that positive, hopeful individuals heal from traumas (both emotional and physical) much more effectively than individuals operating in a state of fear, depression, or anxiety. His remedies are derived from wild flowers and work on mental fixations and emotions that may be damaging the body. Needless to say, Bach flower remedies can contribute to one's overall welfare during detoxification.

BOWEN TECHNIQUE

This gentle, hands-on therapy uses the application of a specific series of physical movements to muscles, tendons, and connective tissue. During detoxification, it can be used to treat aches and pains, as well as more serious injuries or chronic pain that may be partially linked to toxicity. Developed in Australia in the 1950s by Tom Bowen, this therapy has gained worldwide acceptance as a treatment to help heal and regenerate tissues damaged from injury. I have found Bowen Technique extremely effective in alleviating pain and increasing awareness of negative emotions that may be undermining healing efforts. A Bowen session typically lasts forty-five minutes and is performed with the client wearing loose, light clothing.

CRANIO-SACRAL THERAPY

Who would have thought that placing light pressure on the tiny joints of the skull (known as sutures) could contribute to profound healing experiences? William Garner Sutherland, an osteopath in the early twentieth century, discovered that, contrary to what he was taught, the bones of the skull were movable. Although the movement was minute, it was enough to provide relief for patients suffering from diverse ailments. Sutherland further determined that rhythms exist in the cranium and echo fluctuations in the flow of cerebrospinal fluid. When the flow of this fluid is outside its optimal range of ten to fourteen beats or pulses per minute, injury and illness can result. The gentle manipulations to the head and the sacrum (the lower part of the spine) that comprise cranio-sacral therapy can help re-establish the pulse and assist with the healing process.

Cranio-sacral therapy is an excellent, non-invasive adjunct to your detoxification process. A treatment may take sixty to ninety minutes. The manipulations are frequently so delicate that you may wonder whether anything is happening—until after the session. Most cranio-sacral therapists are not medical doctors. Many of these health practitioners have received specialized training at the Upledger Institute, an internationally recognized school founded by American doctor John Upledger.

ENERGY MEDICINE OR ENERGY KINESIOLOGY

Throughout this book, we have learned that everything consists of energy. That includes your body, your thoughts, the chair upon which you sit, the apple you eat and the rocks, flowers, trees, and soil in your garden. Energy is that frequently intangible force that allows us to live. It comes in many forms in our body, including metabolic energy, bioelectrical energy, and biophotonic energy. Despite all these different forms, there are two main energy systems that I focus on. These are best described by two different yet complementary Eastern traditions. Qi (pronounced "chee") forms the basis of the Chinese tradition of energy medicine, including acupuncture. In this system, Qi (or energy) flows through meridians and channels throughout the organs and limbs of the body. Prana is the Indian term for energy. The Pranic system focuses on spirals of energy that travel along the spine and in other locations of the body, where they are referred to as chakras. These two energy systems actually create an excellent illustration of how our bodies are powered. Toxins in their myriad forms can interrupt this flow of energy throughout our bodies, leading to illness and disease.

Energy medicine is a bit of a catch-all category for diverse therapies and practices that use both internal (our own) and external (universal) energy to assist in our healing. Arguably, all healing modalities are energy medicine but the title has become linked to techniques such as acupuncture or acupressure, which focus on alleviating energy blockages in the body, as well as therapies like Reiki and chakra balancing, which introduce additional universal energy into the body.

Energy medicine is also the name of a specific therapy or approach to healing, involving a variety of techniques to balance the body's energy systems, like those you learned earlier in this book. These techniques include touch, specific movements and exercises (not push-ups and sit-ups or what we traditionally refer to as "exercise"), and working in a person's aura. The aura refers to the energetic field that surrounds each of us and actually forms part of our being. Auras have been captured using Kirlian photography techniques. It still amazes me to see the change in the size and strength of a person's aura after they have undergone a positive experience. This could be thinking of a loving relationship, receiving a therapy or treatment from a skilled natural health practitioner, or simply, eating healthy foods or developing a greater connection with his or her life purpose.

Energy medicine is one of the oldest, most powerful forms of medicine known to humankind. In our modern society, however, it can be extremely difficult to find a credible, skilled practitioner. If you do, you will likely encounter an individual who believes that healing must take place on an energetic level before it can be successful at the physical level. Transforming your body at this energetic level will contribute to a successful detoxification experience.

FAR-INFRARED SAUNA THERAPY

From the native civilizations across North America to the Scandinavian cultures of northern Europe, people worldwide have recognized the health benefits of increasing one's body temperature. Unfortunately, sweat lodges are not as common as they once were but modern technology has helped bring the benefits of heat to us in the form of products using far-infrared radiation (FIR). Today, you will find heat lamps, quilts, and even hair dryers that deliver therapeutic heat to our bodies. However, my favourite form of far-infrared radiation technology for the purpose of detoxification is the sauna.

Radiation, you say? Yes, I know radiation has negative connotations in modern society and we avoid all things radioactive (if we know what they are). What most of us do not realize is that radiation comes in many forms. There is the lethal atomic radiation from a nuclear bomb blast. Ultraviolet radiation, such as the harmful rays from the sun, can burn and damage the skin when it penetrates the ozone layers. But the sun also delivers healing, warm rays or radiant heat. This is infrared radiation, a form of energy that heats objects directly. In other words, it does not heat the air in between.

A short science lesson helps to explain the heat/radiation/energy relationship. Infrared radiation is measured as light along the electromagnetic spectrum. It falls below ("infra") the red light segment along this spectrum—hence the name infrared. While it is not visible to the human eye, this light penetrates our skin surface and is absorbed by our cells. Visible light simply bounces off our skin. Near-infrared light is absorbed at the skin level and will cause the surface skin temperature to increase moderately. Far-infrared light can penetrate our bodies up to an estimated four centimetres and works energetically at the cellular level. Research has demonstrated that this penetrating radiant heat can increase metabolism and blood circulation in addition to raising our core body temperature. And what do all of these things have in common? You guessed it: they promote detoxification and help to heal the body.

Please do not confuse FIR saunas with the traditional idea of a sauna. You won't be pouring water over hot rocks to create steam and moist heat. These steam saunas can be beneficial but the high temperatures and humidity can create a cardiovascular risk. FIR saunas mimic nature by delivering radiant heat through ceramic infrared heaters. No hot stones, no water, no humidity, but plenty of sweat. The energy delivered from a FIR sauna creates a "sweat volume" that is two to three times greater than a conventional steam sauna. This is also accomplished at a lower (and therefore less risky) temperature. FIR saunas typically operate in the 110° to 130° F range, while steam saunas can reach 180° to 235° F. Consequently, heart rate and blood pressure concerns are greatly reduced while you sweat out those toxins. The most important thing to remember is to replace that fluid and mineral loss with pure water to prevent dehydration. In addition to your usual eight to ten cups of water daily, add at least two more cups for each sauna session.

If you can find a health practitioner who offers FIR sauna as a therapy, I urge you to consider adding it to the detoxification program. If you can afford to purchase one (about $5,000 and up), it is a great lifestyle addition. These units often look like small cabins constructed of various wood species such as cedar or oak. FIR saunas vary in dimensions but can typically accommodate one to six people.

HOMEOPATHY

What medical substance becomes more powerful when it ceases to exist in its physical form? According to German physician Dr. Samuel Hahnemann, the same substance that potentially causes an illness in the first place. It sounds strange but this is the basic premise of homeopathy: dilute a substance until none of the original material remains and you are left with its "energetic signature."

Hahnemann was not alone in this belief. Hippocrates, the father of modern medicine, stated many centuries ago that "like cures like," and through years of experimentation, Hahnemann discovered that the most effective way to combat particular illnesses was to deliver highly diluted substances to the body that, in their undiluted form, would create the same symptoms of the illness. The word "homeo-pathy" is derived from two Greek words: "homos," meaning like, and "pathos," meaning suffering. If this theory sounds too wacky for you, consider this: that modern, medical marvel known as the vaccine is based on the same principle. Unlike homeopathy, a vaccination will deliver toxic chemical additives such as heavy metals along with the substance intended to help the body.

In my experience, homeopathy is most effective when administered by a skilled practitioner. It is a truly holistic healing modality when a homeopath selects remedies for their physical, emotional, mental, and spiritual attributes. To accomplish such a task, a homeopath may ask you many questions to obtain a clear picture of your symptoms and what conditions make them worse or better. Homeopathic remedies are available in different potencies and dosages, which can be confusing. While there is no single homeopathic remedy to tackle detoxification on an energetic (and ultimately) physical level, a visit to a homeopath may be an interesting addition to your program. You may encounter a powerful healing alternative for specific ailments or issues with which you have been struggling.

LYMPHATIC DRAINAGE

You have now learned how critical proper lymph flow is to good health. You have also learned that unlike the blood in our cardiovascular systems, the lymph system does not have a muscle to pump lymph throughout the body. Our own movements keep lymph flowing.

Fortunately, there is a form of massage that stimulates the network of lymph nodes in our bodies and assists us with toxic elimination. Lymphatic drainage is beneficial for anyone with stagnant lymph and, in our modern world, that is just about everyone. Press firmly under your arms or along your inner thighs. If it is sore to touch, your lymph may be struggling with a toxic buildup. Lymphatic drainage massages use deep, rhythmic, and methodical movements to stretch the tissues in the direction that lymph flows. By stimulating the lymph system, we also stimulate our immune systems to help with healing. This is an excellent addition to a detoxification program, particularly for people who are not capable of exercising or have limited mobility.

MASSAGE

What can I say about massage? When administered by a trained, caring health practitioner, it can be relaxing, revitalizing, and healing all at the same time. It can be your treat for doing such a good job on your detoxification program! The important thing is to find a properly trained therapist with whom you feel comfortable. Keep in mind that there are numerous forms of massage as well: hot stone, Swedish, and Hawaiian, to name a few. Some techniques focus entirely on the physical body while others address emotional and spiritual levels as well. Virtually any form of massage will be of some assistance with cleansing.

NATUROPATHY AND NATURAL MEDICINE

Naturopathy and natural medicine comprise a collection of natural therapies including but not limited to herbalism, nutrition, acupuncture, massage, and homeopathy. Naturopaths or doctors of natural medicine are the doctors who employ some or all of these therapies and healing modalities when they work with a client. Typically, he or she will focus solely on holistic therapies to help a client recover from illness, detoxify, or heal from an injury.

Sessions with a naturopath or a doctor of natural medicine will vary depending on the practitioner's experience and areas of specialization. For example, one person may have a stronger background (and greater success) with herbal remedies, while another may focus more on acupuncture and homeopathy.

OSTEOPATHY

Osteopathy has existed in its modern form since the late nineteenth century, when American doctor and engineer Andrew Taylor Still grew disenchanted with the orthodox approach to medicine. He believed that structural misalignments of the body could lead to illness and injury. By treating the joints, muscles, ligaments, and bones, and improving the client's range of motion, he felt the body could be brought back into a state of balance—in other words, a state of health.

Osteopaths use soft tissue manipulation, massage, and gentle movements of specific joints to help realign the body. This therapy has proven effective for arthritis, asthma, back pain or injuries, bronchitis, bursitis, carpal tunnel syndrome, constipation, earaches, headaches, flu, endometriosis, hearing problems, heartburn, hemorrhoids, menstrual problems, muscle cramps, pain (acute or chronic), prostate problems, sinusitis, sports or traumatic injuries, and varicose veins. Benefits are frequently experienced after a single session but long-term conditions may require multiple visits to the osteopath.

While it may appear from this description that osteopathy is best suited for injuries or postural problems, keep in mind that many of these imbalances are exacerbated by toxicity or are the result of toxic conditions.

QUANTUM BIOFEEDBACK

Quantum biofeedback is high-technology therapy that taps into the primal principles of energy. Based on thirty years of research in the field of bioenergetic medicine, quantum biofeedback detects energetic imbalances in the body by reading the electrical responses of over eight thousand different factors in the body, including pathogens, allergies, hormones, joints, nutrient deficiencies, emotions, and many others. Not only does the device read these energetic frequencies, it assesses them and delivers energetic therapies to the body to help normalize the imbalances.

This is not as far-fetched as it sounds. Science has already proven that everything is energy. It has also determined that each individual thing, whether it is a cell from your lung tissue or a virus, has a unique frequency. Quantum biofeedback devices read these frequencies and search for stress patterns in the body. They then deliver therapies energetically to remind the body of the "correct" or healthy frequency and help the body restore its state of balance. This frequently leads to increased energy, enhanced mental clarity, and improved healing of diverse disorders.

A quantum biofeedback session will vary in length depending on the health concerns of the client and the practitioner's approach. Anywhere from thirty minutes to two hours is common. The biofeedback therapist will place bands around the client's ankles, wrists, and forehead to read the electrical impulses from the body. The whole process is painless but the results can be profound. Quantum biofeedback is an excellent tool for a therapist to uncover specific toxic stresses that may be affecting a person.

REIKI

Reiki is an ancient hands-on healing art that was re-discovered by Mikao Usui in the nineteenth century. A Japanese minister working at a Christian seminary, Usui studied Buddhism, Chinese, and Sanskrit to understand ancient texts on healing. Following a twenty-one-day fast on a mountain, he was struck by a powerful light and saw visions of symbols. These symbols revealed the working of a universal life-force energy as it was described in ancient Sanskrit writings and gave Usui insight into using this energy for the purpose of hands-on healing.

Usui shared this knowledge with sixteen people. Today this gentle, healing modality has spread across the world and is practised by many thousands of people. Reiki (which means universal life force energy) practitioners believe that when energy flow is restored in the body, health is also restored. I believe that scientific testing consistently demonstrates the effectiveness of this form of therapy for a couple of different reasons: our hands emit both electromagnetic energy and infrared light that falls into the healing range of the electromagnetic spectrum (remember the FIR saunas?).

Reiki practitioners will never tell you they are healing you or giving you their energy. They are merely serving as a conduit for universal energy. It is a very caring and generous form of therapy and works on physical, emotional, and spiritual levels. That never hurts when we are looking to restore our health and is especially good for emotional cleansing.

SHIATSU

For those of you who are intrigued with the healing principles of acupuncture but don't like needles, shiatsu, a form of acupressure, may be a good alternative. The word means "finger pressure" in Japanese, which is appropriate for this form of massage. The therapist will use massage techniques to work on the energy meridians within the body.

Shiatsu is an effective technique for releasing toxins from body joints and improving the body's energy flow. These are just two of the many excellent reasons to consider shiatsu during your detoxification program.

THAI MASSAGE

This is another healing modality based on the principles of acupuncture. Also known as Thai yoga massage, this technique is quite a workout for both client and practitioner. It comprises a series of guided stretches and yoga positions to loosen tight muscles, increase flexibility, and disperse energy blockages in the body.

Thai massage is an excellent therapy; however it is quite vigorous. I caution anyone who is considering this form of massage to discuss their current state of health, including injuries or illness, in detail with the practitioner prior to embarking on a session. Thai massage does work on the energy meridians of the body (like acupuncture and yoga) and therefore can offer great benefits during a detoxification program.

Detoxification and healing are most effective when a holistic approach is adopted. That means introducing healing modalities like those described above into a lifestyle that includes nutritious food, clean water, exercise, and a positive outlook on life. Every individual is unique and will respond to healing therapies in a different way. Frequently, we find that we really connect with one form of healing (and certain therapists or health practitioners) over another. I encourage you to explore different forms of therapies and seek out the best experience for you.

In this chapter you learned
  + Many natural healing disciplines support detoxification
  + Some of the best ones are: acupuncture, Alexander Technique, aromatherapy, Bach flower therapy, Bowen Technique, craniosacral, energy medicine or energy kinesiology, far-infrared sauna therapy, homeopathy, lymphatic drainage, massage, naturopathy, osteopathy, quantum biofeedback, Reiki, shiatsu, and Thai yoga massage

References

1. Michelle Schoffro Cook, *Healing Injuries the Natural Way* (Toronto: Your Health Press, 2004).

CHAPTER 13

The Ultimate Body
Detox Plan Recipes

*"The food we put in our systems determines the health of every cell
and organ in our bodies. The human body needs "live" foods
to build "live cells."*
Jay Kordich, "The Juiceman"

In this chapter you will learn
+ How to make delicious cleansing juices and smoothies, including
  ones to detoxify your blood, liver, skin, or to increase healing ability
+ How to prepare herbal teas to purify your blood, liver and
  gallbladder
+ How to make quick salad dressings and salads that are, not
  only delicious, but also lessen inflammation and pain while
  detoxifying your body
+ How to prepare ancient and whole grains
+ How to make delicious cleansing soups and main dishes
+ How to prepare decadent desserts (that still cleanse your body)

JUICES AND SMOOTHIES

Many of the smoothie recipes include frozen banana. I encourage you to peel several bunches of bananas (preferably organic since most conventional bananas are picked green and gas-ripened), set them on a tray, and freeze them. Once they are frozen, put them in a plastic bag and store them in the freezer. When a recipe calls for a frozen banana, simply pull one from your freezer bag as necessary.

Carrot Cleansing Juice

Ginger increases circulation to the muscles in the body, allowing the extra blood and oxygen to fight toxins. It also helps alleviate pain and inflammation. Carrots are an excellent source of beta carotene, which is needed for many detoxification processes.

6 large carrots (remove tops)

1 apple, cored

1 1-inch piece of ginger

Pass all ingredients through a juicer. Drink immediately.

Body Cooler

This is an excellent summertime juice to keep your body cool.

4 carrots

2 celery stalks

1 apple, cored

Juice all ingredients in a juicer. Drink immediately.

Citrus Cleansing Juice

1 orange

1 grapefruit

½ lemon

1 cup water

Juice all citrus ingredients in a citrus juicer. Alternatively, peel and juice in a standard juicer. Add water and drink immediately.

Alkalizing Juice

3 carrots

½ cucumber

½ beet with greens

Juice all ingredients in a juicer. Drink immediately.

Blood, Liver, and Kidney Cleansing Juice

Dandelion is useful for cleansing the blood (which removes toxins from the tissues and joints, thereby speeding healing and reducing pain and inflammation). Be aware that if you drink a fair amount of this juice over a short period of time it can quickly cause a cleansing reaction that initially might produce symptoms like fatigue or headaches. These symptoms will pass as your body becomes "cleaner."

3 apples

handful of fresh dandelion leaves (if you are digging it yourself, be sure to obtain organic dandelion where the land has not been sprayed for several years and is far removed from traffic areas)

Pass all ingredients through a juicer. Drink immediately.

Skin Cleansing Juice

1 cucumber

4 stalks celery

1 to 2 apples (depending on preferred sweetness)

Pass all ingredients through a juicer. Drink immediately.

Enzyme Power Healing Smoothie

Not only is this smoothie delicious and satisfying, it is an amazing healer. Papaya, pineapple, and ripe bananas are loaded with enzymes that help digestion and break down toxins, fat, and inflammation in the body. Bromelain, an enzyme in pineapple, breaks down cholesterol in the blood and reduces inflammation in the blood and tissues. Studies show that it helps to eliminate muscle, joint, and headache pain.[1] Bromelain also helps break down fat. Papain, an enzyme that is plentiful in papaya, breaks down protein molecules in the blood, reducing inflammation that is linked to allergies or pain. Even cancer cells have a protein coating that papain attacks, thereby helping the body deal with these ominous cells. Drink up!

    1 cup chopped papaya
    1 cup chopped fresh pineapple (not canned)
    1 frozen banana

Combine with desired amount of water in a blender and blend to desired smoothie consistency.

Clenzyme Juice

    ½ pineapple, outer skin removed (juice the core as well as the flesh)
    1 1-inch piece of ginger

Pass all ingredients through a juicer. Dilute with pure water to taste. Drink immediately.

Cran-Berry Melon Power Juice

This delectable treat cleanses the urinary tract and the liver, while reducing inflammation in the body. Consider the research behind this delicious drink: cranberries and blueberries line the cells of the urinary tract and bladder, thereby preventing harmful bacteria from anchoring themselves to the cells. Blueberries also contain a powerful anti-inflammatory ingredient that is *ten times* stronger than aspirin (without the harmful side effects). Watermelon is one of the few foods that contain a potent nutraceutical called glutathione. Nutraceuticals are compounds found in food that have nutritional and medicinal properties. This super food greatly improves the Phase 2 detoxification pathway in the liver—a remarkable accomplishment that helps the body more effectively eliminate synthetic chemicals.

2 large slices of watermelon

½ cup blueberries

½ cup cranberries

Push all ingredients through a juicer. Serve over ice if desired.

Banana Nut Shake

2 bananas

4 pitted dates (soaked for at least half an hour)

½ cup almonds

water

Blend all ingredients together until smooth. Add water until desired consistency is reached.

Bobbi's Strawberry Daquiri

1 orange, juiced

1 cup frozen strawberries

½ lime, juiced

Blend all ingredients together until smooth. Drink immediately. Alternatively, peel one orange and half a lime and blend in a blender with frozen strawberries.

HERBAL TEAS

Blood Purifier Tea

This warming tea not only purifies the blood, it lowers cholesterol, urea, and nitrogenous waste products that damage cells. It even cleanses the liver and skin, and soothes the gastrointestinal tract.

Mix the following dried herbs (found in most health food stores) in a jar:

¼ cup peppermint

¼ cup ginger

¼ cup globe artichoke

Add one teaspoon of the mixture (per cup of tea) to a tea strainer or tea ball. Pour boiling water over the tea strainer and let sit for five minutes. Sweeten with one to three drops of stevia per cup (if desired).

Liver/Gallbladder Tea

This tea is also good to help with fat digestion. Many people suffer from headaches because their bodies cannot handle the amount of fat in their diet.

Purchase dried herbs at your local health food store for this recipe. In a jar, mix together the following:

1 part milk thistle seed

1 part artichoke leaves

1 part dandelion root

Use one teaspoon of the herb mixture per cup of water. Simmer in a non-aluminum pot on the stove for fifteen minutes. Strain. Drink one cup of the liquid mixture three times per day.

SALADS AND SALAD DRESSINGS

TIP: For an even higher fibre, higher protein salad, drain a can of beans and add to your favourite salad recipes.

Blueberry Cleansing Salad Dressing

Blueberries are excellent anti-inflammatory agents. They increase the amounts of compounds called heat-shock proteins that decrease as people age, thereby causing inflammation and damage, particularly in the brain. If you blueberries regularly, research shows that these heat-shock proteins stop declining, inflammation decreases, and pain decreases, not to mention that the blueberries just taste fabulous. Blueberries are excellent pain-fighters as well. If toxins in your body are causing pain or inflammation, you'll be happy to learn that blueberries contain a substance that is ten times more potent than aspirin at fighting pain and inflammation.

½ cup blueberries (fresh or frozen)

¾ cup cold-pressed flax seed oil (make sure it is refrigerated)

⅓ cup apple cider vinegar (with sediment in the bottom—purchase at a health food store)

dash of Celtic sea salt (Celtic sea salt is a moist, greyish-coloured salt that contains dozens of minerals, not just sodium. It is not the same as sea salt. I recommend using Celtic sea salt whenever you would normally use salt.)

1 tablespoon pure maple syrup

Blend with a hand mixer or whisk together. If whisking ingredients together, mash the blueberries with a fork. Pour over mixed baby greens since they have the greatest healing properties of various types of lettuce.

Herb Cleansing Salad Dressing

¾ cup cold-pressed flax seed oil (make sure it is refrigerated)

⅓ cup apple cider vinegar (with sediment in the bottom—purchase at a health food store)

½ teaspoon Celtic sea salt

½ teaspoon basil

½ teaspoon thyme

½ teaspoon oregano

dash of cayenne pepper

Whisk all ingredients together. Or place in a jar and shake well. Pour over fresh mesclun salad greens (mixed baby greens).

Miso Vinaigrette

⅔ cup cold-pressed organic canola oil

1/3 cup rice vinegar

2 heaping teaspoons red miso

1 level teaspoon honey

Shake all ingredients together in a jar or blend with a hand blender. Toss with greens.

Raw Spa Wild Berry Dressing

I borrowed this delicious salad dressing recipe from The Raw Spa Kitchen.

½ cup mixed berries, fresh or frozen

1 to 2 tablespoons of honey

1 tablespoon extra virgin olive oil

3 tablespoons fresh lemon juice

1 tablespoon orange juice

Blend the ingredients and pour on your favourite salad greens.

Mom's Coleslaw

½ cabbage, grated

2 carrots, grated

¼ onion, finely grated or chopped

1 stalk celery, finely chopped

½ cup organic raisins

1 apple, grated (optional)

Dressing:

½ cup extra virgin olive oil

3 tablespoons unpasteurized honey

¼ cup unpasteurized apple cider vinegar

Mix all coleslaw ingredients together in a bowl. In a jar, mix together dressing ingredients and shake until blended. Pour dressing over coleslaw until well mixed. Serve.

Healing 5-Bean Salad

I have another name for this recipe: "the power pusher." You'll discover why within a day or so of eating it.

1 can cooked mixed beans (such as kidney, garbanzo, pinto, etc.), rinsed

2 stalks celery, finely chopped

¼ purple onion, finely chopped

½ green pepper, finely chopped

½ red pepper, finely chopped

1 green onion, finely chopped

¾ cup cold-pressed flax seed oil (make sure it is refrigerated)

⅓ cup apple cider vinegar (with sediment in the bottom—purchase at a health food store)

½ teaspoon Celtic sea salt

1 tablespoon pure maple syrup

½ teaspoon basil

½ teaspoon thyme

½ teaspoon oregano

dash of cayenne pepper

Mix the cooked beans and chopped vegetables together in a bowl. In a jar, whisk together the flax seed oil, apple cider vinegar, Celtic sea salt, maple syrup, basil, thyme, oregano, and cayenne pepper. Pour half of the dressing over the bean and vegetable mixture. For the best taste, let it marinate overnight or for a couple of hours. Store the remaining dressing in a covered jar in the refrigerator for later use.

Mexican Salad

1 head of leaf or romaine lettuce, washed and dried

1 tomato, chopped into cubes

1 avocado, chopped into cubes

dash Celtic sea salt

handful fresh cilantro

1 tablespoon cold-pressed flax oil

1 lime

1 small clove garlic

Cut or tear the lettuce and place it in bowls to form a base for the other salad ingredients. Put tomato, avocado, Celtic sea salt, cilantro, and flax oil together in a separate bowl. Squeeze the juice of the lime over the tomato-avocado mixture. Chop or press garlic and add it to the tomato-avocado mixture. Toss ingredients together. Serve the tomato-avocado mixture over the salad greens.

Sweet Broccoli Salad

My sister developed this recipe to find a delicious way to get raw broccoli into her diet.

1 head of broccoli, chopped finely

1 carrot, grated

2 apples, cored and chopped

1 cup raisins (soak in water for at least half an hour before using, then drain and discard water)

¼ cup raw, unsalted sunflower seeds

Mix all the ingredients together.

Dressing:

½ cup extra-virgin oil or Udo's Special Blend oil

1 tablespoon unpasteurized apple cider vinegar

1 tablespoon unpasteurized honey

Mix the dressing ingredients together. Pour on vegetable mixture. Toss and enjoy.

Bobbi's Complete Salad

1 head of romaine lettuce, cleaned and chopped into bite-sized pieces

1 avocado, cubed

1 tomato, chopped

½ red onion, sliced into thin rings

½ red pepper, chopped

Dressing:

½ cup extra-virgin olive oil

2 tablespoons unpasteurized apple cider vinegar

1 teaspoon organic balsamic vinegar

1 tablespoon unpasteurized honey

1 teaspoon crushed garlic, basil, oregano, or your favourite herb
(optional)

Blend all the dressing ingredients together. Divide the salad ingredients into bowls. Pour the dressing over the salad. Serve.

Spinach Salad

1 small package baby spinach leaves

¼ cup raw, unsalted walnut pieces

1 avocado, peeled, pitted, and chopped

2 hardboiled eggs, peeled and sliced (optional)

Dressing:

¼ cup cold-pressed walnut oil

⅛ cup organic balsamic vinegar

1 teaspoon pure maple syrup

Mix all the dressing ingredients together. Toss over spinach leaves.
Place the dressed greens in serving bowls. Top with walnuts, avocado,
and hardboiled eggs (if using). Serve.

Bobbi's Zesty Salad

1 grapefruit, peeled and cut into sections

1 orange, peeled and cut into sections

1 avocado, peeled, pitted, and chopped

½ red onion, chopped finely

2 cups bean sprouts (washed and drained)

Mix all salad ingredients together.

Dressing:

¾ cup extra-virgin olive oil

¼ cup organic red wine vinegar

½ teaspoon dried oregano

½ teaspoon chilli powder

¼ teaspoon black pepper

¼ teaspoon crushed chillies (optional)

Mix all the dressing ingredients together. Pour the desired amount over the salad ingredients.

Asian Rice Salad

½ cup almonds, chopped and soaked in water overnight (discard water after soaking)

2 cups cooked brown or wild rice

¾ cup chopped celery

¾ cup chopped red pepper

1 green onion, chopped

large handful of fresh parsley, chopped

Mix all ingredients together.

Dressing:

¼ cup extra-virgin olive oil or Udo's Special Blend oil

½ tablespoons wheat-free tamari (available at most health food stores)

dash Celtic sea salt

Mix the dressing ingredients together. Pour over salad ingredients and toss.

Italian Pasta Salad

Bobbi-Jo Meyer created this healthy alternative to a traditional pasta salad.

3 cups cooked pasta (brown rice, spelt, or kamut)

1 ½cups chopped broccoli florets

1 tomato, chopped

1 scallion, minced

1 carrot, thinly sliced

Dressing:

2 teaspoons dried oregano

1 tablespoon dried parsley

¼ cup extra-virgin olive oil

3 tablespoons organic balsamic vinegar

2 tablespoons unpasteurized apple cider vinegar

Mix all the salad ingredients together in a large bowl. Mix all the dressing ingredients in a jar. Shake and pour over salad. Serve.

ENTRÉES

When you're cooking, never allow oil to get so hot it smokes. The temperature at which an oil will smoke varies from one kind of oil to another. The smoke temperature is the point at which the heat chemically alters the oil, making it no longer healthy to consume. It is far better to use a lower temperature when cooking with oils and take a few extra minutes than to destroy the health properties of the meal from overheating.

Some of the entrée recipes call for cooked whole grains. Here is a chart for cooking them. The amount of water is per cup of grain.

Grain	Amount of Water	Cooking Time	Special Directions
Amaranth	2 ½ to 3 cups	20 to 25 minutes	
Barley (Pearl)	2 ½ to 3 cups	50 to 55 minutes	
Millet	2 ½ cups	35 to 40 minutes	Best if toasted first
Oat	3 to 4 cups	45 to 60 minutes	Best if soaked overnight
Oats (rolled)	1 ½ cups	10 minutes	Stir oats into boiling water
Quinoa	1 cup	15 minutes	Best if toasted first
Brown Rice	2 ¼ cups	35 to 40 minutes	

When using legumes, be sure to drain and rinse them thoroughly. This helps to prevent the flatulence commonly associated with legumes.

Lentil Dahl

This Indian curry tastes so fabulous you may forget you are on a cleansing regime. This healing food stabilizes blood sugar, cleanses the intestinal tract, protects the liver from toxins, lowers cholesterol, and reduces joint inflammation. It is also quick and easy to make. It is one of my favourites.

1 yam, cubed

2 tablespoons extra-virgin olive oil

1 large onion, chopped

½ teaspoon mustard seeds

4 dried red chillies

1 1-inch piece of ginger, grated

2 cloves garlic, chopped

3 cups cooked lentils (or two small cans, rinsed)

½ teaspoon turmeric

1 teaspoon Celtic sea salt

fresh cilantro (if desired)

½ cup water

In a medium to large pot, boil the cubed yam in water until soft. Pour off excess water, leaving enough to mash the yam with a hand blender until smooth. In a frying pan, cook the onion, mustard seeds, chillies, ginger, and garlic in the olive oil over low heat until the onion is transparent. Add the onion mixture to the mashed yam. Then add the lentils, turmeric, Celtic sea salt and ½ cup water. Stir together. Let the mixture simmer over low heat until warmed and the flavours mingle. Serve in bowls with fresh cilantro as a garnish.

Italian White Bean Stew

1 small onion, chopped

1 clove garlic, chopped

2 tablespoons extra-virgin olive oil

½ bunch spinach, chopped coarsely

4 medium tomatoes, chopped
1 can lima beans or other white beans, drained and rinsed
chopped basil for garnish
Celtic sea salt to taste

In a large skillet, sauté the onion and garlic in olive oil over low heat until translucent. Add the spinach, tomatoes, and lima beans. Stir. Cook uncovered for about 10 minutes or until the tomatoes and spinach are cooked and the stew has thickened. Add the chopped basil and Celtic sea salt and stir. Serve.

Hot and Sour Soup

This is one of the easiest soups to make, but don't let its simplicity fool you. It is a meal in a bowl (or pot depending on how you choose to serve it).

Broth:
1 medium onion, chopped
4 teaspoons freshly grated ginger (approximately 1 1-inch piece of ginger)
1 small dried chili
2 tablespoons extra-virgin olive oil
8 cups of water
2 tablespoons apple cider vinegar
5 tablespoons low-sodium tamari or soy sauce
small handful of dried arame (seaweed) strips, or one small piece of dried kelp
juice of 1 lemon

In a medium-sized pot, sauté the onion, ginger, and chilli in 1 tablespoon of olive oil until the onion is transparent. Add water and all additional ingredients and let simmer for 10 to 30 minutes (depending on the time available). Longer simmering allows the flavours to mingle.

Hot and Sour Hotpot Variation

To the above broth, add the following:

> grated carrots
>
> 1 handful of rice vermicelli noodles
>
> thinly sliced red and green peppers
>
> thinly sliced button mushrooms
>
> 1 green onion, sliced diagonally
>
> cilantro, finely chopped
>
> ⅔ cup cubed tofu

In a serving pot or several bowls, arrange the hot pot ingredients in small clusters. When ready to serve, pour the broth over the hot pot ingredients and let sit for several minutes.

Zesty Tomato Soup

Here is another simple, but fabulous, recipe from The Raw Spa Kitchen.

> 1 cup tomatoes
>
> ¾ cup water
>
> 3 tablespoons olive oil
>
> ½ teaspoon Celtic sea salt
>
> ½ teaspoon thyme
>
> ½ teaspoon dill
>
> 2 cloves garlic
>
> ¼ teaspoon black pepper

Blend all the ingredients in a blender and serve.

Roasted Vegetable and Rosemary Soup

This is my husband's all-time favourite soup. You may forget how detoxifying it really is while you are enjoying the savoury taste. It is packed with cleansing veggies and nutritious extra-virgin olive oil.

> Vegetables:
>
> 1 sweet potato or yam

1 red pepper

1 green pepper

2 medium-sized potatoes

1 large onion

5 cloves garlic

1 carrot

Marinade:

3 tablespoons of extra-virgin olive oil

1 sprig of fresh rosemary or 2 teaspoons of dried rosemary

1 teaspoon thyme (dried)

½ teaspoon Celtic sea salt.

Mix all the marinade ingredients together.

Chop all the vegetables (excluding the garlic) into medium-sized pieces. Put all the vegetables in a large bowl. Toss them with the marinade until coated. You may need to do this in two stages, depending on the size of the bowl you are using. Spread all the vegetables on a large baking tray. Bake at 350 degrees F for 1 hour or until vegetables are soft. Purée in a food processor or blender, adding hot water or stock to thin to desired consistency. Serve. Add Celtic sea salt to taste.

Moroccan Vegetable and Wild Rice Soup

Don't let the ingredient list fool you. This is a quick and easy recipe to make, especially if you use the slicing blade of a food processor. The result is a rich and hearty soup that is almost a stew and is loaded with cleansing vegetables and fibre.

3 tablespoons extra-virgin olive oil

4 cloves garlic, chopped

1 large onion, chopped

8 cups water

½ cup wild rice

1 sweet potato, chopped

2 stalks celery

2 carrots, chopped

4 small red-skinned potatoes, sliced

½ cup frozen peas

3 teaspoons cinnamon

½ teaspoon allspice

1 teaspoon molasses

2 teaspoons Celtic sea salt (or to taste)

¼ teaspoon garlic powder

2 teaspoons cumin

dash of cayenne pepper

1 red pepper, sliced

½ cup cooked kidney or pinto beans

In a large pot, sauté the garlic cloves and onion in the olive oil. When the garlic and onions are slightly browned, add the water, wild rice, sweet potato, celery, carrots, potatoes, peas, cinnamon, allspice, molasses, Celtic sea salt, garlic powder, cumin, and dash of cayenne pepper. Bring to a boil. Once the water begins boiling, turn down the heat and let simmer for 45 minutes. Add the red pepper and kidney or pinto beans and simmer for an additional 15 minutes or longer, until the vegetables are cooked and the wild rice is soft. Simmer longer, if desired to allow flavours to mingle. Stir any spices that sit at the top of the pot into the broth before serving.

Jewelled Moroccan Stew

2 tablespoons olive oil

1 onion, finely chopped

3 cloves garlic, finely chopped

1 teaspoon fresh ginger, chopped

1 teaspoon ground tumeric

2 teaspoons ground cumin

½ teaspoon dried hot pepper flakes

3 medium tomatoes diced

1 13-ounce can chick peas, drained and rinsed

½ cup golden raisins (be sure they are organic and do not contain sulphites)

1 cup water

½ medium butternut squash, peeled and cut into cubes

1 red pepper, cut into 1-inch pieces

Heat the olive oil in a large saucepan. Add the onion and sauté until translucent. Add the spices and cook for 1 minute. Add the remaining ingredients and bring to a boil, then reduce the heat and simmer for 40 minutes (with lid on). Serve on its own or with rice or couscous.

APPETIZERS, SNACKS, AND SPREADS

Stuffed Celery Sticks

celery, cleaned and cut into 3-inch pieces

raw almond butter

Spread almond butter on the concave part of the celery.

Mom's Omega-3 Almond Butter

3 cups of raw almonds

½ cup of cold-pressed flax oil

Put the raw almonds into a food processor bowl and start to chop. While chopping, slowly drizzle ½ cup of the flax oil into the nuts. Blend until almond butter reaches the desired level of smoothness.

Bobbi's Mexican Sandwich Spread

½ green pepper, minced

½ red pepper, minced

½ stalk celery, minced

2 small scallions, minced (or use one green onion, chopped)

juice of 1 lemon (use fresh lemon juice only)

dash of chili powder

dash of cumin powder

dash of cayenne powder

1 avocado, peeled and pitted

Mix all ingredients, mashing the avocado into the vegetables and spices. Serve on whole grain pitas, tortillas, and wrap. Alternatively, serve on toasted whole-grain spelt or kamut bread or buns.

If desired, add either of the following:

Baby spinach leaves

Sliced tomatoes

Celery Seed Bread

Brush olive oil on slices of whole-grain bread (preferably 100 percent whole-grain spelt or kamut) and sprinkle with celery seeds. Bake in a 350 degree F oven until golden-brown and serve as a tasty side dish. Celery seeds contain more than 20 anti-inflammatory compounds and help cleanse the kidneys and urinary tract.

BREAD AND PANCAKES

Quick Spelt Bread

1 ¾ cup whole-grain spelt flour

½ cup multi-grain cereal

1 ½ teaspoons baking powder (make sure it is aluminum-free)

2 tablespoons water

1 ¼ cup soy milk, rice milk, or almond milk

2 tablespoons honey

¼ cup canola oil (cold-pressed organic preferably)

2 tablespoons ground flax seeds (or grind your own in a coffee grinder)

Mix the flour, cereal, and baking powder together in a food processor or mixer. In a separate bowl, whisk liquid ingredients together with the ground flax seeds. Slowly pour the wet ingredients into the dry ingredients. Pour into a greased loaf pan and bake at 350 degrees F for 50 to 55 minutes.

Apple Pancakes

¾ cup kamut or spelt flour

1 teaspoon aluminum-free baking powder

½ teaspoon Celtic sea salt (be sure it is finely ground)

1 cup soy milk, rice milk, or almond milk

½ teaspoon cinnamon

1 apple, sliced

Mix all ingredients (except apples) together. Cook by scoopfuls in an oiled frying pan. While the first side is cooking, push the apple slices into the batter. When golden brown, flip and cook the other side. Serve immediately.

DESSERTS

Berry Blast Ice Cream

Ice cream on a cleansing program? you may be asking yourself. Cleansing does not mean starvation, nor does it mean deprivation. This ice cream contains powerful natural phytochemicals that help diminish inflammation in the organs and tissues of your body while cleansing the lymphatic system. It is best to eat this ice cream on an empty stomach, as part of your morning fruit regime, or about three hours after eating later in the day.

1 cup frozen raspberries

1 cup frozen blueberries

2 frozen bananas

Blend all the ingredients in a food processor or push through a Champion juicer with the blank screen. Eat immediately.

Mixed Berry Pie

Crust:

1 cup rolled oats

½ cup almonds

1 teaspoon cinnamon

pinch of Celtic sea salt

1 cup spelt, kamut, or whole-grain flour

⅓ cup cold-pressed organic canola oil

¼ cup maple syrup.

In a food processor, grind oats, almonds, cinnamon, and salt. Stir the flour into the oats mixture. Finally, add the oil and maple syrup and mix to form a soft dough. Press into an oiled and floured 10-inch pie plate and flute the edges if desired. Bake at 350 degrees F for 25 minutes or until golden-coloured. Allow to cool while preparing filling.

Filling:

¼ cup agar flakes (a form of tasteless seaweed that is packed with nutrients and serves as a thickener)

2 cups of unsweetened raspberry, strawberry, mixed berry, or apple juice

⅓ cup arrowroot

¼ cup maple syrup

4 cups fresh or frozen mixed berries of your choice

Mix agar flakes and juice together in a saucepan and bring to a rolling boil. Let cook, uncovered for 2 to 3 minutes after it starts boiling, stirring constantly. In a small bowl, whisk together the arrowroot and maple syrup. Add to the juice mixture and whisk constantly, until thickened. Stir the berries into the mixture and pour immediately into the pie crust. Refrigerate for 1 to 2 hours or until set.

Coconut Nut Balls

My sister, Bobbi-Jo, founder of The Raw Spa Kitchen in southern Ontario, created this delicious, nutritious, and high-fibre recipe.

1 cup raw, unsalted almonds or walnuts, ground

1 cup unsweetened coconut flakes

1 cup raw almond butter

2 tablespoons pure maple syrup (not the "maple-like" products on the market)

additional ground nuts or coconut

Mix all the ingredients, except additional ground nuts or coconut, together in a food processor. Form into small balls and roll in the ground nuts or coconut.

Bobbi's Orange Date and Nut Balls

1 cup raw, unsalted pecans

½ cup chopped dates (without pits)

½ cup raisins (be sure they are unsulphured)

1 ½ tablespoons grated orange rind

Mix all ingredients together in a food processor. Form into balls about.

Berry "Gelatin"

Typically jelly is made from gelatin (which is an animal product). This gelatin recipe is made with mineral-rich agar, which is a type of seaweed. Now you can have your minerals and your gelatin too.

¼ cup agar flakes (available in most health food stores)

2 cups of raspberry or apple juice

2 tablespoons of maple syrup (optional)

⅓ cup arrowroot

4 cups fresh or frozen berries

In a saucepan, mix together the agar and juice with a whisk. Bring to a boil on high heat, whisking the entire time. When the juice starts boiling, lower the heat to medium and continue cooking for 2 to 3 minutes to dissolve the agar. In a separate bowl, mix the maple syrup and arrowroot together until well blended. If you opt not to use the maple syrup, mix the arrowroot with 2 tablespoons of water. Add the maple syrup-arrowroot mixture to the agar mixture in the saucepan. Whisk until thick (approximately 1 minute). Remove from heat, add the berries, and pour into individual glass or ceramic serving cups. Refrigerate for 1 to 2 hours to set.

Thumbprints

These cookies are not suitable for regular consumption during *The 4-Week Ultimate Body Detox Plan*, but they are excellent as an occasional sweet that still helps you maintain the many benefits of the detox program after you have completed it. Full of fibre and minerals, these decadent cookies taste great and are nutritious too. If that weren't enough, they are simple to make.

> 1 cup of almonds
> 1 cup rolled oats
> 1 ¼ cups of oat, kamut, spelt, or rice flour
> 1 teaspoon cinnamon
> ½ cup maple syrup
> ½ cup cold-pressed walnut oil
> ½ cup unsweetened raspberry or strawberry jam

Preheat oven to 350 degrees F. Grind the almonds and oats to a fine meal in a food processor. Add the flour, cinnamon, maple syrup, and oil to the almonds-oat mixture and process until well combined. Oil a cookie sheet. Form the dough into walnut-sized balls. Place them on the cookie sheet. Press an indentation in the centre of each ball with your thumb. Fill the indentation with jam. Continue until all dough has been used. Bake for 10 to 15 minutes or until golden. Makes approximately 24 cookies.

Wild Berry Crumble

My sister developed this recipe as part of her Raw Spa Kitchen workshops. It is a simple, delicious, and healthy alternative to cooked berry crumbles. By keeping the fruit raw, this recipe has an alkalizing effect on the body. Cooking fruit has an acidifying effect on your body.

Base:

1 cup oats

½ cup almonds

¼ teaspoon cinnamon

3 tablespoons unpasteurized honey

Combine the above ingredients in a food processor. Process until mixed, but still slightly coarse. Divide evenly among small dessert bowls (approximately four).

Fruit Filling:

2 cups mixed berries, frozen or fresh

Divide the fruit among the four dessert bowls, placing it on top of the oat-almond mixture.

Sauce:

½ cup unsweetened juice (apple, pear, or another of your choice)

1 tablespoon arrowroot powder (available in most health food stores)

Combine the juice and arrowroot in a small saucepan. Bring to boil, stirring constantly, until mixture thickens. Pour over the fruit. Refrigerate until set (1 to 2 hours) and serve. Alternatively, make this dessert the day before serving.

Mom's Tropical Fruit Salad

½ pineapple, inner stem and outer skin removed, pulp chopped into bite-sized pieces

3+1 oranges: peel and cut 3 oranges into bite-sized sections, reserve 1 orange

½ cup shredded, unsweetened coconut

½ cup raw, unsalted pecans or almonds

Mix all the ingredients except one orange together in a bowl. Squeeze the remaining orange over the fruit salad and mix again. Serve immediately.

Shortcake Balls

1 cup unsweetened oat flakes or oatmeal

½ cup dates, pitted

⅓ cup unsweetened shredded coconut

1 teaspoon pure vanilla extract (not artificial vanilla)

1 tablespoon unpasteurized honey or pure maple syrup

Mix all the ingredients in a food processor for 2 minutes or until well combined. Roll into small walnut-sized balls. Store in a covered container in the refrigerator. They will last about one week.

References

1. Kathi Keville, *Herbs for Chronic Fatigue* (New Canaan, CT: Keats Publishing, Inc., 1998), pp. 50, 54.

CHAPTER 14

The 4-Week Ultimate Body Detox Plan Lifestyle

Life is no brief candle to me. It is sort of a splendid torch which I have got hold of for the moment, and I want to make it burn as brightly as possible before handing it on to future generations.... I want to be thoroughly used up before I die.
This is the true joy of my life.... Being used for a purpose recognized by yourself as a mighty one, being a force of nature... instead of a feverish, selfish little clod of ailments and grievances, complaining that the world will not devote itself to making you happy.

George Bernard Shaw

Congratulations! By now you have likely completed *The 4-Week Ultimate Body Detox Plan*. You are probably experiencing greater energy, improved health, freedom from negative symptoms, and an increased sense of vitality. If not, you may wish to return to Chapters 7 through 11 to target your cleansing efforts on the appropriate detox organs and emotions discussed earlier.

If you have chronic health problems, you may need to conduct more extensive cleansing. Follow the many suggestions in this book. You may also wish to seek assistance from a skilled detoxification therapist.

I have witnessed people transformed beyond their wildest dreams using the power of detoxification, done properly and thoroughly. I am one of these people. Detoxification, using the principles and practices suggested in *The 4-Week Ultimate Body Detox Plan*, gave me my life back. Whenever I sense some negative symptoms creeping up again, I start detoxifying and begin to feel immediate improvements. Everyone eats poorly sometimes. When you do, recognize that you have a powerful tool in *The 4-Week Ultimate Body Detox Plan* to help you get back on track. That does not mean you should abuse your body with harmful foods and beverages, stress, and toxic environments only to rely on detoxification to "get you out of trouble."

On the contrary, what you do on a regular basis is the most important factor in having great health, not what you do occasionally. You learned some wonderful health habits over the last four weeks, such as juicing, eating more raw foods, taking green food supplements, exercising regularly, drinking lemon water in the morning, meditation and breathing techniques, emotional cleansing techniques, and some powerful energy medicine tools. I urge you to make these habits part of your regular lifestyle. The return on this simple investment in your time and energy will be great. Your body will thank you with greater resistance to disease, improved energy and vitality, and an overall feeling of well-being.

Remember, when it comes to health, you are as good as what you are putting into your body, whether it is processed food or organic, natural foods. The computer term GIGO—garbage in, garbage out—really does apply to your health as well. Forget the search for the miracle pill. Take control of your life by eating well, exercising, taking time out to rest, improving your energies, and limiting your future exposure to toxins. Stop envying people who seem to have it all: great health, great looks, and joie de vivre. Join their ranks by continuing what you have learned in *The 4-Week Ultimate Body Detox Plan*.

Schedule time in your agenda throughout the year to follow the program again. Make it a part of your life.

Life is for living fully. There is only one person who can create the best life imaginable for you—you. You have many great tools for creating the life you've imagined—go confidently in the direction of your dreams. I wish you health and happiness.

Resources

ABOUT THE AUTHOR

Michelle Schoffro Cook, DNM, DAc, CNC, CITP, is a Doctor of
Natural Medicine, Doctor of Acupuncture, Holistic Life Coach®,
Biofeedback Therapist, Holistic Nutritionist, Energy Medicine Practitioner, Reconnective™ Healing Practitioner, and Reiki Master. She
is the Director of Healing Body, Mind & Spirit® —a holistic health
and wellness centre in Western Canada. Dr. Michelle Schoffro
Cook's regular columns appear in the popular health magazines,
Health 'N Vitality, Beyond Fitness, and *Natural Living*. She has contributed over 200 articles to more than 50 magazines, journals, and
newspapers worldwide. Your Health Press released Dr. Schoffro
Cook's second book, *Healing Injuries the Natural Way*, in early 2004
(www.healinginjuries.com). She is the recipient of the prestigious
Forty Under 40 Award as one of the top business people and lead-
ers in Canada's Capital Region under the age of forty. Dr. Schoffro
Cook has also received four communications and writing awards
for her work. She works and lives with her husband in beautiful
Western Canada.

For more information about Michelle Schoffro Cook and her work,
visit her Web site: www.energyeffect.com.

Cellfood®

Cellfood® is a unique cell-oxygenating liquid formula that delivers 78 trace minerals and elements, 34 enzymes, 17 amino acids, and electrolytes and utilizes a unique water-splitting technology to release abundant oxygen into the body. It is readily absorbed by the body at the cellular level, making a wealth of nutrients available to your cells for optimum healing. Unlike other oxygen products I've tried, Cellfood® delivers the oxygen slowly, thereby preventing free radical damage. Cellfood® also helps normalize an acidic pH of the body, which is integral to proper detoxification and healing. It also assists with energy and boosts the immune system. I recommend taking eight drops of Cellfood® three times per day in a glass of pure water. In addition to oxygen, it contains the following essential nutrients:

1. **Trace Minerals and Elements**: actinium, antimony, argon, astatine, barium, beryllium, bismuth, boron, bromine, calcium, carbon, cerium, cesium, chromium, cobalt, copper, dysprosium, erbium, europium, fluorine, gadolinium, gallium, germanium, gold, hafnium, helium, holmium, hydrogen, indium, iodine, iridium, iron, krypton, lanthanum, lithium, lutetium, magnesium, manganese, molybdenum, neodymium, neon, nickel, niobium, nitrogen, osmium, oxygen, palladium, phosphorous, platinum, polonium, potassium, praseodymium, promethium, rhenium, rhodium, rubidium, ruthenium, samarium, selenium, silica, silicon, silver, sodium, sulfur, tantalum, technetium, tellurium, terbium, thallium, thorium, tin, titanium, tungsten, vanadium, xenon, ytterbium, zinc, and zirconium (does not contain aluminium, cadmium, chlorine, mercury, lead, or radium.)

2. **Metabolic Enzymes**: hydrolases, carbohydrases: maltase, sucrase, emulsin nucleases: polynucleotidase, nucleotidase; hydrases: fumarase, enolase; peptidases: aminopolypeptidase, dipeptidase, prolinase; copper enzymes: tyrosinase, ascorbic

acid oxidase; esterase: lipase, phosphotase, sulfatase; iron enzymes: catalase, cytochrome oxidase, peroxidase; enzymes containing coenzymes 1 and/or 2: lactic dehydrogenase, robison ester dehydrogenase; yellow enzymes: Warburg's yellow enzymes, diaphorase, Haas enzyme, cytochrome C reductase; enzymes which reduce cytochrome: succinic dehydrogenase; aidase: urease; mutases: aldehyde mutase, glyoxalase; desmolases: zymohexase, carboxylase; and other enzymes: phosphorylase, phosphohexisomerase, hexokinase, phosphoglumutase

3. **Amino Acids**: alanine, arginine, aspartic acid, cystine, glutamic acid, glycine, histidine, isoleucine, lysine, methionine, phenylalanine, proline, serine, threonine, tryptophan, tyrosine, valine.

Cellfood® is available from most health food stores and healthcare practitioners. For more information, I recommend Lumina Health Products at www.luminahealth.com. You can contact them by calling 1-800-749-9196 or e-mailing to info@luminahealth.com.

ENERGY MEDICINE

For more information on the energy medicine techniques presented in this book or a wealth of other powerful energy techniques, consult Donna Eden and David Feinstein. *Energy Medicine*. New York: Jeremy P. Tarcher/Penguin, 1998.

Donna Eden also has an excellent three-part video series called *Energy Healing with Donna Eden*. Both the book and the video series are available from www.innersource.net.
1-800-835-8332

LYMPHATIC SYSTEM

For more information about the lymphatic system and its connection to pain, inflammation, excessive weight and disorders like fibromyalgia, lupus, and chronic fatigue syndrome, I recommend Harvey Diamond's books:

Fit for Life not Fat for Life
The Fit for Life Solution
The Fibromyalgia / Lupus / Chronic Fatigue Syndrome Connection
www.fitforlifetime.com
1-877-335-1509

NATURAL CLEANING PRODUCTS

If you are looking for cleaning products that kill bacteria without exposing you or your loved ones to toxins, here are several brands of natural cleaning products:

Seventh Generation
Nature Clean
Orange TKO
Citrisolve

They are available in most health food stores and many grocery stores.

NUTRITIONAL CHELATION

Nutritional chelation is a powerful therapy that involves no harsh chemicals or invasive equipment. Instead, high doses of particular nutrients help to dissolve plaque on arterial walls and bind to heavy metals. It has been used successfully in cases of atherosclerosis to avoid bypass surgery. For more information, I recommend David W. Rowland's book, *The Nutritional Bypass: Reverse Atherosclerosis Without Surgery, Revised Edition 1999.* Parry Sound, ON: Rowland Publications, 1999.
www.rowlandpub.com
705-746-1086

PAIN-RELATED CONCERNS

For more information on pain-related health concerns, traumatic or sports injuries, fibromyalgia, arthritis, or osteoporosis, see my earlier book, *Healing Injuries the Natural Way: How to Mend Bones, Muscles, Tendons and More*. It is available from Trafford Publishing at 1-888-232-4444 or online at www.healinginjuries.com or www.energyeffect.com.

QUAIL EGG HOMOGENATE

French researcher J. C. Truffier proved the beneficial effects of quail eggs on allergy symptoms. Additional clinical trials show that sublingual tablets of quail egg homogenate are effective against allergic asthma, seasonal rhinitis, and allergic rhinitis due to dust mites. They are available from some holistic health professionals or visit www.energyeffect.com.

QUANTUM BIOFEEDBACK

Developed by a former NASA engineer over the last several decades, quantum biofeedback determines stress patterns in the body on over 8,000 different items: organs, bones, muscles, hormones, emotional states, energy meridians, viruses, bacteria, foods (and related sensitivities), and much more. In addition to detecting stressors, it also emits healthy patterns back to your body to help it restore health. The process is painless and relaxing. It combines ancient healing wisdom with modern technology for a therapy that is truly the best of both worlds. For more information, visit www.energyeffect.com.

Bibliography

Baillie-Hamilton, Paula. *The Body Restoration Plan*. New York, NY: Avery, 2003.

Barnes, Kathleen. "The little fiber pill that can detox your whole body." *Woman's World*. April 27, 2004.

Boyle, Jillian. "Is Lymphatic Stress the Reason You're Fat? Bloated? Hungry for Junk Food?" *Woman's World*. March 2, 2004.

"Brain Scans, Blood Tests Show Positive Effects of Meditation." *Health Behavior News Service*. August 16, 2003.

Cook, Michelle. "Harness the power of love." *Ottawa Citizen*. Ottawa, February 14, 2001.

Cook, Michelle. "How do You Spell Relief—Drugs or Natural Remedies?" *Health 'N Vitality*, February 2002.

Cook, Michelle. "Is your lawn worth your health?" *The Ottawa Citizen*. June 5, 2001.

Crawford, Leslie. "Containing Plastics" *Alternative Medicine* February 2004.

"Detoxification" Informational Brochure. Advanced Nutrition Publications, Inc., 1994.

Diamond, Harvey. *The Fit for Life Solution*. St. Paul, MN: Dragon Door Publications, Inc., 2002.

Eden, Donna and Feinstein, David. *Energy Medicine*. Jeremy P. Tarcher/Penguin, New York: 1998.

Erickson, Kim. "On the Fast Track," *Herbs for Health*, March/April 2004.

Fitzgerald, Patricia. *The Detox Solution*. Santa Monica, CA: Illumination Press, 2001.

Foster, Helen. Detox Solutions. Octopus Publishing Group, Ltd., UK, 2004.

Gang Sha, MD, Zhi. *Power Healing*. SanFrancisco, CA: HarperCollins Publishers, Inc., 2002.

Gerber, MD, Richard. *Vibrational Medicine for the 21st Century: The Complete Guide to Energy Healing and Spiritual Transformation*. New York, NY: Eagle Brook, 2000.

Gilbere, ND, DAHom, PhD, Gloria. "A Doctor's Solution to 'Plumbing Problems,' In Your Gut That Is!" *Total Health*. Volume 26, No. 1.

Gittleman, MS, CNS, Ann Louise. *The Fat Flush Plan*. New York, NY: McGraw-Hill, 2002.

Gursche, Siegfried. *Good Fats and Oils*. Vancouver, BC: Alive Books.

Henderson, Paul. "Neem and Catnip Oil Repels Mosquitoes Best." *Vitality Magazine*.

Htut, Tin. "The Effects of Meditation on the Body." *Triplegem.plus.com*. September 18, 1999.

Keville, Kathi. *Herbs for Chronic Fatigue*. New Canaan, CT: Keats Publishing, Inc., 1998.

Krohn, MD, Jacqueline and Taylor, MA, Frances. *Natural Detoxification: A Practical Encyclopedia*. Vancouver, BC: Hartley & Marks Publishers, Inc., 2000.

Krop, MD, FAAEM, Jozef J. *Healing the Planet One Patient at a Time*. Alton, ON: KOS Publishing, Inc. 2002.

Muir, Maya. "Ridding the Body of Toxic Chemicals: Detoxification Protocols," *Alternative & Complementary Therapies*. August 1998.

Murray, ND, Michael. "Good Health and Optimism Go Hand in Hand" *Health & Wellness Newsletter*. Spring 2004.

Root, MD, MPH, David E. and Anderson, Joan. "Reducing Toxic Body Burdens Advancing in Innovative Technique," *Occupational Health and Safety News Digest #2*, April, 1986.

Rowland, PhD, David W., *The Nutritional Bypass*. Rowland Publications, Parry Sound, Ontario: 1999.

Schoffro Cook, Michelle, "The Secret of Great Health—an Interview with Best-Selling Author Harvey Diamond," April 2003.

Schoffro Cook, Michelle. "Home Sweet Home," *Health 'N Vitality*.

Schoffro Cook, DNM, DAc, CNC, CITP, Michelle. *Healing Injuries the Natural Way*. Toronto, ON: Your Health Press, 2004.

Schoffro Cook, DNM, DAc, CNC, Michelle. "Digestion Tips that Aren't Hard to Swallow." *Natural Living Magazine*.

Simester, Lisha. *The Natural Health Bible*. North Vancouver: Whitecap Books, 2001.

"The Importance of Detoxification" Informational Brochure. Advanced Nutrition Publications, Inc., 2002.

Williams, Xandria. *The Herbal Detox Plan*. Carlsbad, CA: Hay House, 2004.

Young, Ph.D., D.Sc, Robert O. and Redford Young, Shelley *The pH Miracle: Balance Your Diet, Reclaim Your Health*.

Index

B

baby products, 55
Bach, Edward, 173, 273
Bach flower therapy, 173–176, 273
Baillie-Hamilton, Paula, 76
balmony (*Chelone glabra*), 239
bananas, 122
barbecuing, health risks of, 35
barberry (*Berberis vulgaris*), 239–240
basin, tub and tile cleaner, 64
bayberry, 237
beans, 232
bearberry (*Arctostaphylos Uva ursi*), 186
beauty products, 52–58, 108–110
beets, 122–123, 229
benzene, 66
Berkeley Wellness Letter, 75
beta carotene, 102, 233
beverages
    alcohol, 33
    coffee, 31–33
    plastic in, 33–35
    water, 37–39
Bifidobacterium, 128
bilberries, 258
bile, 90, 222, 237, 238, 240, 241
bilirubin, 226
birch (*Betula pendula*), 186–187
bisphenol-A (BPA), 34
black root (*Leptandra virginica*), 240
bladder. *See* Phase 1: kidneys,
    urinary tract and intestinal tract
bleach, 64
bleached products, 32, 56
bloated tissues, 96
blocked absorption of nutrients, 91
blood, 139–141, 250–252
    see also Phase 4: blood, lungs
    and skin
Blood and Circulatory System
    Stress Quiz, 253
blood-brain barrier, 30–31
blood-lungs-skin cleansing tea
    blend, 140

blood purifier, 264
blood purifier tea, 290–291
bloodstream, 96–97
blue flag (*Iris versicolor*), 240
blueberries, 123, 258
the body
    detoxification mechanisms,
        22–23
        see also detoxification organs
    elimination of toxins, 75–76
    meridians in, 150
    needs of, 11
    as a vehicle, 23
body fat
    air pollution and, 51
    and pesticides, 29
    synthetic chemicals and, 50
    and toxins, 12, 76
boldo (*Peumus boldo*), 185, 240–241
borage, 261
bowel movements, 90, 240, 241
bowels, 137–138
    see also Phase 1: kidneys,
        urinary tract and intestinal tract
Bowen, Tom, 274
Bowen Technique, 274
bread, spelt, 305–306
breast cancer, and pesticide and
    fertilizer use, 70
breast disease, 192
breast milk, 71–72
breathing
    dangers of, 50
        see also air pollution
    homes, 58–62, 64–69
    industrial airborne chemicals,
        71–73
    personal hygiene products,
        52–58
    smoking, 51–52
breathing exercises, 260
breathing meditation, 170
broccoli, 230
bronchial asthma, 262, 263

bronchial spasms and coughs, 262, 263
bronchitis, 256, 260, 261, 263
buchu (*Agathosma betulina*), 186
burdock, 240, 266
burning urination, 186

C

cabbage, 123
caffeine, 31–33, 195
caffeylquinic acids, 237
calcium, 101, 102, 103, 258
Canadian Institute of Child Health, 70
cancer, 256
    see also carcinogens
candida, 197–200, 240
candida cleansing, 201
Candida Quiz, 199–200
candidiasis, 197
carbon monoxide, 73
carcinogens
    in baby products, 55
    barbequing, and benzopyrene, 35
    chlorine in water, 37
    in feminine products, 56
    fluoride, 38
    in food, 30
    formaldehyde, 52–58, 61
    in hair dyes, 55–56
    pesticides and, 28
    in plastic, 34
    synthetic colours, 54
    in toothpaste, 56
cardiovascular exercise, 255
cardiovascular system, 96–97
carnitine, 232
carpet shampoos, 61, 64
carrier oil, 147
carrots, 123, 229
Castleman, Michael, 242
catarrh, 217, 260, 262, 264
catnip, as mosquito repellant, 55
cayenne, 232
celebration of success, 163
celery, 123, 187

celery seed (*Apium groweolens*), 123, 187
Cellfood, 116, 127, 128, 134, 136, 141, 315–316
cellulase, 233
cellulite, 130, 138
    see also Phase 2: lymphatic system (and cellulite)
cellulose, 254
The Cellute Solution (Dancey), 210
Celtic sea salt, 120
Center for Conservative Therapy, 88
Centers for Disease Control and Prevention (CDC), 34
chakras, 275
channels. *See* meridian
cherries, 123–124
chewing food, 194
chi, 270
children
    of smoking parents, 52
    susceptibility to toxins, 12
chlorine, 37, 59, 66
chlorophyll, 128, 139, 212, 258
cholecystitis, 240
cholesterol, 251, 252
chronic fatigue syndrome, 223–224
cinnamon, 233
circulatory system, 250–252
cirrhosis of the liver, 33
citric acid, 212
Clean and Healthy Home Quiz, 62–64
cleaning products, 58–62, 64–69, 107–108, 119
cleansing. *See* detoxification
cleansing herbal teas, 147–149
    see also herbal tea blends
cleansing order, 85, 223
cleavers (*Galium aparine*), 185, 216, 267
coal tar colours, 55–56
coffee, 31–33
cold-pressed oils, 134
colic, 239
colitis, 203, 261

detoxification
  see also Ultimate Body Detox Plan
  benefits of, 13, 14–15
  described, 6
  effectiveness of, 87–89
  experimentation with approaches, 8
  vs. fasting, 86
  healing power of, 6–7
  natural detoxification mecha-
    nisms, 22–23
  nutrient requirements, 87,
    100–104
  and nutritional status, 98–99
  order of cleansing, 85, 223
  process of, 85–89
  rate of detoxification, 98–100, 115
  short-term, 88
  side effects of, 85
  stages of, 15–16
  various programs, effect of, 84
detoxification organs
  bloodstream, 96–97
  cardiovascular system, 96–97
  digestive system, 90–94
  fatty deposits and, 97
  lungs, 94–95
  lymphatic system, 95–96
  respiratory system, 94–95
  skin, 94
Diamond, Harvey, 39–40, 95
diarrhea, 203, 261
diazolidinyl urea, 52–58, 56
diet. See North American diet
dietanolamine (DEA), 53
digestion, 190–192, 194
digestive difficulties. See indigestion
digestive enzyme, 127, 139, 196, 233
digestive system
  gallbladder, 92
  intestinal tract, 90–91
  kidneys, 92–94
  liver, 92
  urinary tract, 92–94
digestive tract, 90–91

dinners, 134–135
dioxin, 32, 56
Director of your life, 160
Discover, 100
disease, and toxins, 21–23, 76–77
dishwashing detergent, 64
dishwashing liquid, 64
disinfectants, 60, 61, 64
diuretic, herbal, 185
DNA, and thoughts, 47–48
drain cleaner, 64
drugs
  pharmaceutical.
    See pharmaceutical drugs
  recreational drugs, 52
  side effects, 40
Duke, James, 187, 238
Dunne, Brenda, 46
dysentery, 202, 255
dyspepsia, 239

E
echinacea, 216
eczema, 240
Eden, Donna, 154, 172, 218, 264
eggs
  organic, 213, 231
  quail eggs, 259–260
Einstein, Albert, 153, 154
elecampane (Inula helenium),
  261–262
electrical signals, 128–129
emotional detox principles
  attitude shifts, 161
  celebration of success, 163
  getting what you give out, 164
  keep on trucking, 165
  others' successes, 163
  self-honesty, 161
  self-nurturance, 161
  self-respect, 161
  sharing your success, 164
  supportive and positive people,
    163–164

far-infrared radiation (FIR) sauna
    therapy, 276–278
farmed fish, 30
fasting, *vs.* detoxification, 86
fat-fighting foods, 231–233
The Fat Flush Plan (Gittleman), 96,
    210, 237
fat-soluble chemicals, 222–226
fats
    animal fats, 230
    hydrogenated, 35–37
    hydrogenated fats, 119
    trans fats, 35–37
fatty acid deficiencies, 225
fatty deposits, 97, 138–139
    see also Phase 3: liver and gall-
    bladder (and fatty deposits)
fatty foods, 230
"feel-good" hormones, 20
Feinstein, David, 154, 172, 218, 264
feminine products, 56
fertilizer, 70–71
fever, 217, 261
fibrocystic breast disease, 217
fibromyalgia, 223–224
fish, farmed, 30
Fit for Life (Diamond), 39–40, 95
Fitzgerald, Patricia, 28, 31, 32, 35,
    37, 53, 71, 72
flavonoids, 212, 254, 258–259
flax seeds and flax seed oil, 124, 196,
    213, 229–230, 233, 254, 258
floor polish, 65
flora supplement, 128
flower therapy, Bach, 173–176
fluid consumption during meals,
    194–195, 229
fluid retention, 186, 211, 241
fluoride, 38, 56
folate, 254
folic acid, 102
food allergies and sensitivities,
    29–30
food colouring, 30–31

food poisoning, 203
food processing
    avoiding, 119
    chemicals, addition of, 29
    effects of, 26, 27
food sources of vitamins and minerals,
    102–104
foods
    artificial sweeteners, 26–27
    barbecuing, 35
    to be avoided, 120–121
    for blood, 253–254
    for circulatory system, 253–254
    and constipation, 196
    cooked foods, 183
    to eat, 121
    essential fatty acids, 213–214
    farmed fish, 30
    fat-fighting foods, 231–233
    fresh foods, 119
    fried foods, 119
    for gallbladder, 228–233
    hydrogenated fats, 35–37
    imported foods, and DDT, 29
    for intestinal tract, 194–200
    for kidneys, 183–184
    for liver, 228–233
    for lungs, 257–259
    for lymphatic system, 211–214
    magnesium in, 201–202
    MSG, 31
    optimum cleansing foods, 121–126
    organic foods, 116
    pesticides, herbicides and fungicides,
        28–30
    in Phase 1: kidneys and bowels,
        183–184, 194–200
    in Phase 2: lymphatic system
        (and cellulite), 211–214
    in Phase 3: liver and gallbladder
        (and fatty deposits), 228–233
    in Phase 4: blood, lungs and
        skin, 253–254, 257–259, 266
    plastic in, 33–35

liver congestion, 240
liver-gallbladder tea blend, 139, 291
liver problems, 261
liver swelling, 237
liver tea blend, 238
lobelia (*Lobelia inflata*), 262, 263
Love and Survival (Ornish), 48–49
low-fat diets, 225
lunches, 133–134
Lung and Respiratory System Stress
    Quiz, 257
lung disorders, 262
lungs, 94–95, 139–141, 256–257
    see also Phase 4: blood, lungs
    and skin
lungwort (*Pulmonaria officinalis*), 263
lycopene, 232
lye, 68
lymph fluid, 208–209
lymph-stimulating bath, 146
Lymph Stress Quiz, 209–210
lymphatic drainage, 279
lymphatic massage, 147
lymphatic system
    see also Phase 2: lymphatic
        system (and cellulite)
    deficiencies, 210
    described, 208–209
    as detoxification mechanism,
        95–96
    Phase 2, 138
    physical activity, need for, 21
    resources, 317–318
lymphatic tea blend, 138

M

magic programs, 85–86
magnesium, 104, 201–202
malaria, 240
malic acid, 212, 231
maltase, 233
maneb, 70
manganese, 104
margarine, 36, 119

marshmallow root (*Althaea
    officinalis*), 203
massage
    described, 280
    for lung cleansing, 264–265
    lymphatic massage, 147
    neurolymphatic massage points,
        218, 219, 234
    Phase 2: lymphatic system (and
    cellulite), 214
    Phase 3: liver and gallbladder
    (and fatty deposits), 234, 244–245
    Phase 4: blood, lungs and skin,
        147, 264–265
    Thai massage, 283
mastitis, 217
meats, 116–117, 196
medicines, 9, 22, 39–41
meditation, 166, 170–172
menstrual bloating, 187
menstruation, 203
meridian, 94, 150–151
metabolism, slowed, 225
methyl, 56
Meyer, Bobbi-Jo, 297, 307–308
milk thistle seed supplement, 139
milk thistle (*Silybum marianum*),
    235–236, 237, 242
minerals, 100, 103–104
mini-trampoline, 118, 130–131
Minnesota Multiphasic Personality
    Inventory (MMPI), 158
miracle pills, 85–86
*Molecules of Emotion: The Science
    Behind Mind-Body Medicine*
    (Pert), 172
molybdenum, 104
mornings, 130–133
mosquito repellants, 55
mould and mildew cleaners, 61, 65
mouth, 90
MSG, 31
mucilage, 203
mucus, excess, 261, 263, 264

mullein (*Verbascum thapsus*), 262, 263
multivitamin and mineral, 127, 234
mumps, 217

spelt bread, 305–306
spinach salad, 296
strawberry daiquiri, 290
stuffed celery sticks, 304
sweet broccoli salad, 295
thumbprints, 309
tomato soup, 301
tropical fruit salad, 310
zesty salad, 296–297
recreational drugs, 52, 118
red clover (*Trifolium pratense*), 264
reducing your exposure to toxins,
    106–110, 114
refined carbohydrates, 230
refined sugar. *See* sugar
regulatory process, 62
reiki, 282–283
Rein, Glen, 47
respect for yourself, 161
respiratory problems, chronic, 264
respiratory system, 94–95, 256–257
    see also Phase 4: blood, lungs
        and skin
rheumatism, 186–187, 217, 237, 261
rhubarb root (*Rheum officinale*), 203
riboflavin, 103
Rigden, Scott, 223–224
rivers, 38–39
Rowland, David, 252

S
saccharin, 26–27
safety studies, lack of, 61–62
salad dressing recipes
    berry dressing, raw spa wild, 293
    blueberry cleansing salad
        dressing, 291–292
    herb cleansing salad dressing, 292
    miso vinaigrette, 293
salad dressings, 134
salad ingredients, 134–135
salads
    Asian rice salad, 297
    bean salad (5-bean), 294

coleslaw, 293
complete salad, 295–296
Italian pasta salad, 297–298
Mexican salad, 294–295
spinach salad, 296
sweet broccoli salad, 295
zesty salad, 296–297
salespeople, 180
salivary glands, 90
salmon, 30
salt, 120, 252
salt intake, 183
sanitary pads, 56
sauna, 277
scented products, 54–55
scouring powder (chlorinated), 65
seafood, 196
seaweed, 125–126
second-hand smoke, 69
sedative properties, 241
seeds, 213–214
Segerstrom, Suzanne, 162
selenium, 104
self-honesty, 161
self-love, 49
self-respect, 161
senior citizens, and prescription
    drugs, 40
Sha, Zhi Gang, 168
sharing your success, 164
shiatsu, 283
short-term detoxification, 88
shortening, 37
Silver Birch, 186–187
silver polish, 65
silybin, 236
silymarin, 235–236
sinusitis, 259
skin
    see also Phase 4: blood, lungs
        and skin
    cleansing the, 139–141
    described, 265
    as detoxification mechanism, 94

typical North American diet. *See*
North American diet